Off Target

Other Books by Jill Ammon Vanderwood

The San Francisco Adventures of Sara the Pineapple Cat

Through the Rug Tenth Anniversary Edition

Through the Rug 2: Follow that Dog Tenth Anniversary Edition

Through the Rug 3: Charm Forest;

What's It Like, Living Green? Kids Teaching Kids, by the Way They Live

Santa's Mysterious Boot

The Year Santa Lost His List

Drugs Make You Un-Smarter

Shaking Behind the Microphone: Overcoming the Fear of Public Speaking

Erase the Problem of Bullying

Off Target

The Path You Choose – #1

Jill Ammon Vanderwood

Illustrated by Kerah Diez and Trevor Brown

IC
PRESS
Idea Creations Press
www.ideacreationspress.com

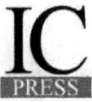

IC
PRESS
Idea Creations Press
www.ideacreationspress.com

This book was the creation of the author Jill Ammon Vanderwood as Off Target: The Path You Choose Book 1, and has no connection with any other similar book series where the reader makes a choice.

978-1-948804-08-0

Publisher's Catalog-In-Publishing Data

Vanderwood, Jill Ammon, author
Off Target / Jill Ammon Vanderwood
First trade paperback original edition. | Salt Lake City: Idea Creations Press, 2019.
ISBN 978-1-948804-08-0 | LCCN 2019930685
The Path You Choose / Gun Violence | BISAC: Young Adult Fiction > School & Education / Young Adult Fiction > General

Printed in the U. S. A

Dedication

This book is dedicated to students who have the courage to stand up and report threats to their school and to the student survivor activists of Marjorie Stoneman Douglas High School, who are fighting for change in gun laws.

Acknowledgements

I would like to thank my husband, Bill Vanderwood; Kathy and Doug Jones at Idea Creations Press; the conceal and carry instructors at Smith and Edwards, in Utah; Judge Tom Jacobs from Askajudge.com; Damion Bosco from Justanswer.com and the Gifford Law Center to Prevent Gun Violence.

Story Guide

Story one: <u>You take the Gun—Trevor finds out about the gun:</u> picture 1, 2 picture, 3, 4, 5 picture, 6, 9, 11, 13, 14 picture, 15, 21, ending page 24.

Story two: <u>You take the gun home</u>— picture 1, 2 picture, 3, 4, 5 picture 6, 9, 11, 13, 19, 25, 26, 28, ending page 29, see picture page 35.

Story three: <u>You plan to come back for target practice—You tell your parents about the gun,</u> picture 1, 2 picture, 3, 4, 5 picture, 6, 10, 12, 17, 31, 34, 35 picture, 36, 37, ending page 40.

Story four: <u>You have something else to do,</u> picture, 1, 2 picture, 5 picture, 6, 10, 12, 17, 30, 38, 39, 47, 62, 63, 64 picture, 65, 70, ending page 71.

Story five: <u>Six Kids, One Gun—You leave with Trevor:</u> picture, 1, 2 picture, 3, 4, 5 picture, 6, 10, 12, 17, 27, 44, 45 picture 46, 51, 52, 53 picture, 59, 60, 62, 63, 64 picture, 65, 70, ending page 71.

Story six: <u>Six Kids, One Gun—You don't tell anyone for about an hour</u>—picture, 1, 2 picture, 3, 4, 5 picture, 6, 10, 12, 17, 27, 44, 45 picture, 46, 51, 52, 53 picture, 57, 58, ending page 61 * see picture page 64.

Story seven: <u>Six Kids, One Gun—You stay and call 911</u>—picture, 1, 2 picture 3, 4, 5 picture, 6, 10, 12, 17, 27, 44, 45 picture, 46, 51, 54, 66, 67, 68, 69, 73, <u>74</u> picture, 75, ending page 76

Story eight: <u>Target Practice—You take your turn to shoot the gun:</u> Picture, 1, 2 picture, 3, 4, 5 picture, 6, 10, 12, 17, 27, 43, 77, 85, 86 picture, 87. You turn yourself in continue with pages: 90, 92, 93, 95, 100, 101, 103, 104, ending on page 106 with a picture on page 107.

Story nine: <u>Target Practice—You hide at Eric's house</u>—picture 1, 2, 3, 4, 5 picture, 6, 10, 12, 27, 43, 77, 85, 86 picture, 87, 88, 89, 98, 99, 102, ending page 105, * picture page 107.

Story ten: <u>Target Practice—You refuse to shoot the gun:</u> picture, 1, 2 picture, 3, 5 picture, 6, 10, 12, 27, 43, 77, 82, 91, ending on page 94.

Story eleven: <u>Hide and seek</u>—picture, 1, 2, 3, 4, 5 picture, 6, 10, 12, 27, 56, 83, 96 picture, 97, 108, 109, ending page 110.

Story twelve: <u>You think Eric might take the gun to school—Something just doesn't feel right:</u> picture, 1, 2 picture, 3, 4, 5 picture, 6, 7, 8, 16, 18, 20, 22 picture, 23, 32, 33 ending on page 41.

Story thirteen: <u>You think Eric might take a gun to school—You talk to a counselor about Eric:</u> picture, 1, 2 picture, 3, 4, 5 picture, 6, 7, 8, 16, 18, 42, 48 picture, 49, 50, 55, 72, ending on page 78, picture on page 79.

Story fourteen: <u>You think Eric might take a gun to school—Eric takes the gun to school:</u> picture 1, 2 picture, 3, 5 picture, 7, 8, 16, 18, 80 picture, 81, ending on page 84.

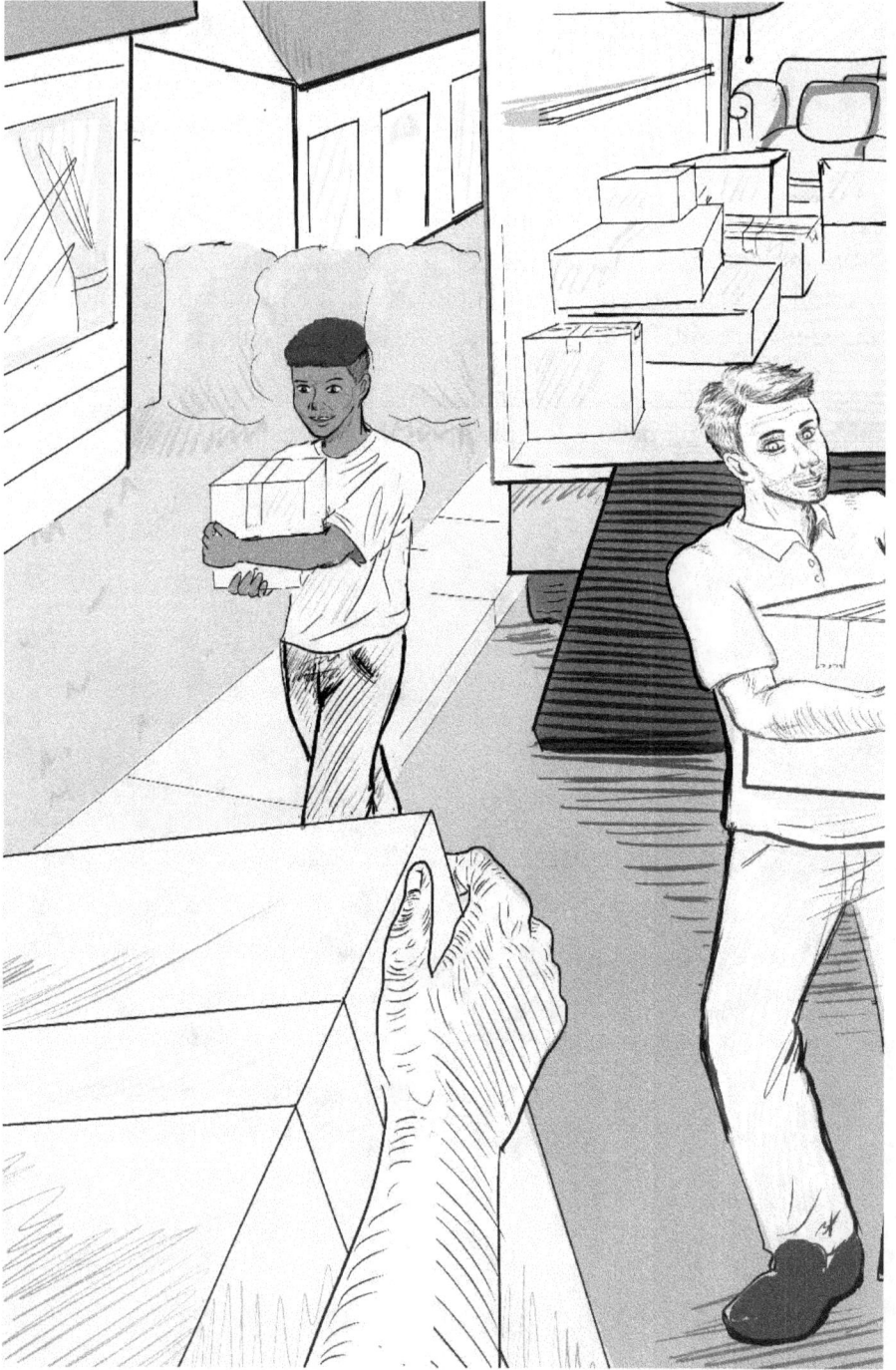

Your dad got a job in a different state and your family is moving from the town where you've lived since Kindergarten. You leave all your friends behind and the house where you lived for your whole life; where you marked your growth chart on the closet wall.

Your family will now live in a city where you only know your grandparents and a few older cousins. You're nervous about starting over in a new school.

When your dad pulls into the driveway with the large U-Haul® truck, a neighbor comes over, bringing his son to help unload the truck.

"Hi, I'm Trevor," You find out that he's your age and he tells you, "Since you're new in school, I'll help you find your way around and introduce you to some of my friends."

You feel very relieved knowing you won't have to enter the new school alone.

Continue on page 3.

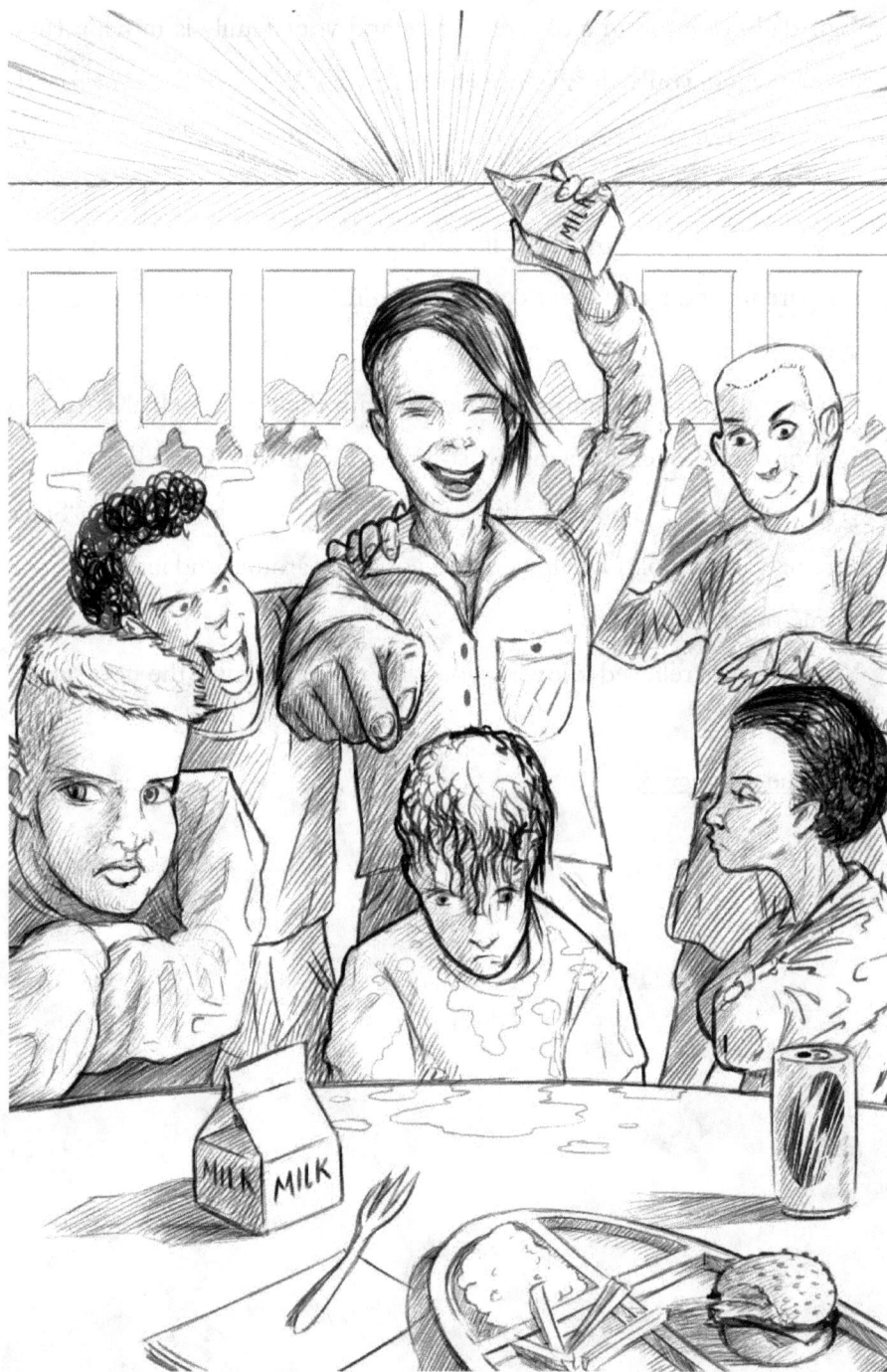

Your new friend Trevor is true to his word and shows you around the school, helps you find your locker and shows you the way to each classroom throughout the day. You eat together at lunch.

"Hey," Trevor says, "I want to introduce you to my friends. "This is Eric, and Tyler." Each of the guys wave a hand, so you'll know who they are.

Eric says, "Welcome to our school."

You say, "Thanks!"

Trevor continues, "And this is Sara and Lisa." The girls' wave and say, "Hi".

While you're having lunch together, a group of three larger guys come up to the table. One of the guys tells Eric to back off from his girlfriend. He then pours milk over Eric's head. Trevor and Tyler stand up, ready to fight these guys, but Eric shakes his head, telling them to stay out of it.

"Hey, new kid," the bully points to you, "You've really picked a group of losers," he says before the group walks away.

Eric is so mad, he makes a fist and says some threatening words, while everyone in your group takes their napkin and helps him wipe off the milk dripping from his head and down his chin.

Continue on Page 4.

After your first day of school, Trevor brings you along to his friend Eric's house where the same friendly kids you met at lunch, often gather after school. There are no parents around. You play football outside with your new friends and then everyone goes inside for snacks. Eric says to the group, "Hey, I want to show you something." He motions for all of you to follow him.

You, along with the group of three guys and two girls follow Eric upstairs to his parent's bedroom. Eric opens the drawer on his mother's nightstand to show a gun.

"My mom keeps this loaded in case someone breaks into the house. This handgun has sixteen rounds in the clip. None of the bullets have been fired."

Eric also shows the group where she keeps the clips for the weapon. Each of you "ooh and aww" and wait your turn to touch the gun.

Tyler says, "Eric, you should take this gun to school. No one would mess with you if you had a gun."

You hear Trevor gasp and say, "No, no, no," under his breath.

"Yeah! That's called crowd control," Lisa says.

Continue on page 6.

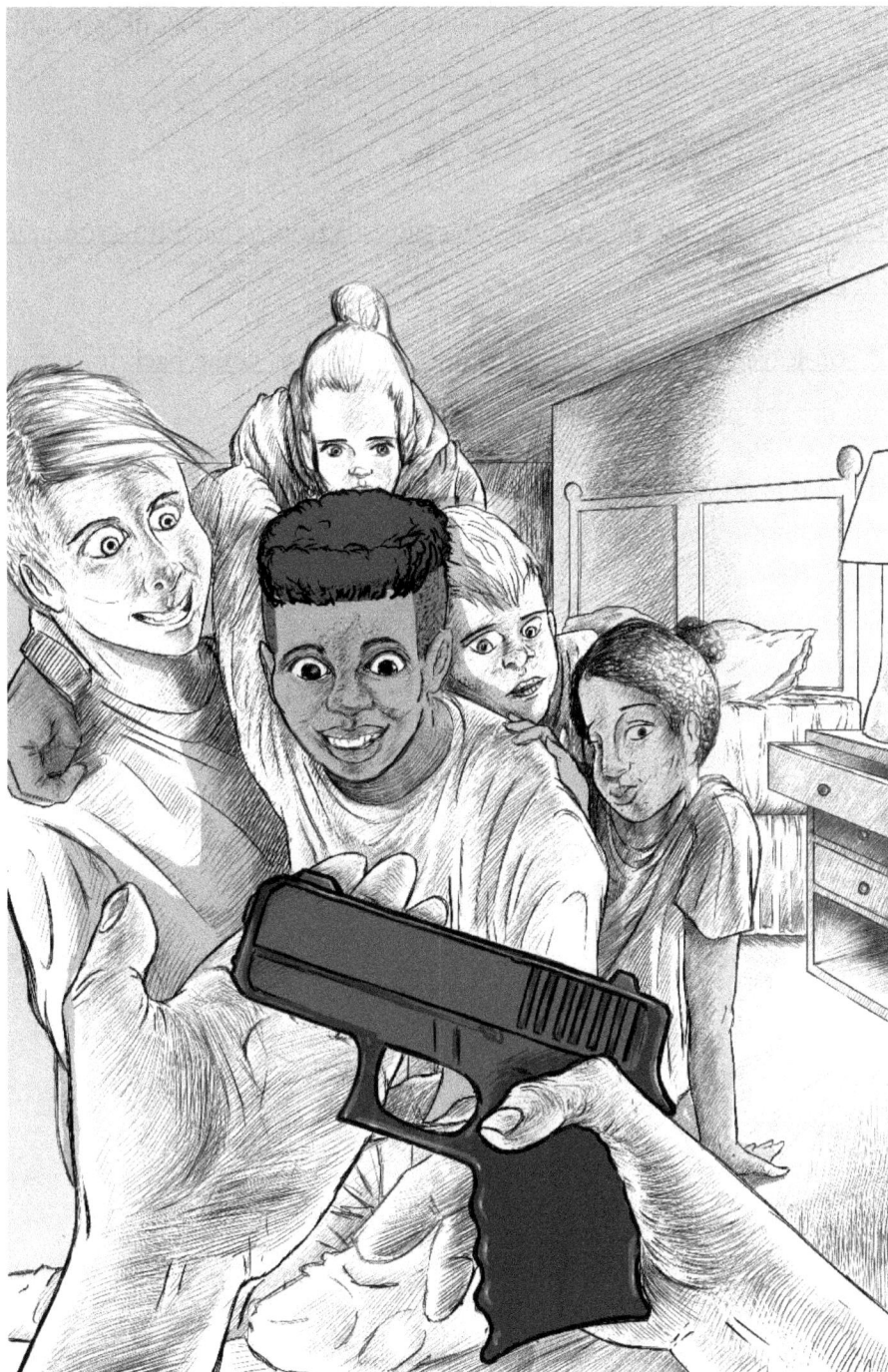

Trevor says, "I think it's cool to hold the gun, but if someone got shot, this weapon would have our fingerprints all over it."

What should you do? It's time to choose a path:

If you decide to take the gun to prevent anyone from being hurt—continue on page 9.

If you leave the house with the others and plan to come back for target practice the next day--continue on page 10.

If you're worried that Eric will take the gun to school—continue on page 7.

If you're worried that Eric will take the gun to school:

You're the last person to hold the gun, being careful not to touch the trigger. This is the first time you've ever seen a gun up close. It's a handgun, and you wonder what kind of damage this weapon could do if it went off. In the movies and on TV, people get shot all the time, but they probably use fake blood and fake bullets. This is too real.

When Eric gets the gun back, he puts his finger on the trigger and pretends to shoot, aiming at different targets around the room and making the sound of shooting. "Pow, pow, pow!" Everyone ducks. You close your eyes and suck in a breath, worried about what could happen.

You're relieved when Eric carefully puts the gun back into the drawer and closes it. The group leaves the bedroom and goes downstairs.

You leave the house with Trevor. On the way home, Trevor tells you about the guys who used to be friends with Eric. Now they bully him every chance they get. "If you think the incident today at lunchtime was bad, it's nothing compared to the way they treated him last year. The worst thing is that we all used to be friends."

Continue on page 8.

"I thought it must be bad, the way they pushed him around at school today," you say. "You don't really think Eric will take the gun to school, do you?"

"No, I don't." Trevor says. "Someone else suggested that he take the gun to school. That wasn't Eric's idea. I know Eric very well and I didn't hear anything about it from him."

When you get home, you say goodbye to Trevor and plan to walk to school together the next day.

You didn't hear Eric say that he would take a gun to school, did you?

Thoughts go around and around in your head. You have a hard time concentrating on your homework. When it comes to dinner, you pick at your food. The things you're telling your parents about school and your new group of friends, don't reflect the truth about what you're really feeling.

You feel trapped. You don't know what it's like to have old friends turn on you the way they turned on Eric. You don't want to be a troublemaker after your first day at a new school.

Continue on page 16.

If you decide to take the gun to prevent anyone from being hurt:

After each person has a turn holding the gun, you're filled with fear. You're the new kid and worry about speaking up. When someone suggests that Eric should take the gun to school to deal with the bullies, the fear takes over and you feel you need to do something to stop him.

When Eric gets the gun back, he puts his finger on the trigger and pretends to shoot, aiming at different targets around the room, and making the sound of shooting. "Pow, pow, pow!" Everyone ducks. You close your eyes and suck in a breath, worried about what could happen.

You're relieved when Eric carefully puts the gun back into the drawer and closes it.

Now's your chance to make a real difference. A plan is forming in your head. You feel that you should act on it.

When everyone leaves the room, you fake needing to use the bathroom. Eric shows you to the room down the hall.

You come out of the bathroom and listen to hear if the other kids are downstairs. You can hear voices near the front door. It's time to make your move.

Continue on page 11.

If you leave the house with the others and plan to come back for target practice the next day

You're the last person to hold the gun, being careful not to touch the trigger. This is the first time you've ever seen a gun up close. This is a handgun and you wonder what kind of damage this weapon could do if it went off. In the movies and on TV people get shot all the time, but they probably use fake blood and fake bullets. This is too real.

When Eric gets the gun back, he puts his finger on the trigger and pretends to shoot, aiming at different targets around the room, and making the sound of shooting. "Pow, pow, pow!" Everyone ducks. You close your eyes and suck in a breath, worried about what could happen.

You're relieved when Eric carefully puts the gun back into the drawer and closes it. The group leaves the upstairs bedroom and goes downstairs. Continue on page 12.

Sneaking back into the parent's room, you slowly open the drawer to the nightstand. Taking a few tissues from a box on the stand, you pick up the handgun and slip it into your backpack.

You then leave the room, close the bedroom door and walk down the steps to join the others. Now you're sure that Eric won't take the gun to school or put anyone in danger.

You leave the house with Trevor. On the way home, Trevor tells you that Eric *is* a good guy. "He used to play on the football team until a group of jocks started picking on him. He now does everything he can to avoid this group of bullies." According to Trevor, what you saw at lunch time when one of the bullies poured milk on Eric's head was nothing compared to the other things that have been going on since last school year.

"Really, what could be worse?" you ask.

Trevor tells you, "Last year they put itching powder in his football uniform. After that, they took his helmet, so he couldn't play with the team. This year the guys have gone into a central computer to change his grades to failing.

Continue on page 13.

You and Trevor say goodbye to the others and leave the house together. On the way home, Trevor tells you, "Eric *is* a good guy. He used to play on the football team until a group of jocks started picking on him. He now does everything he can to avoid this group of bullies." According to Trevor, what you saw at lunchtime when one of the bullies poured milk on Eric's head was nothing compared to the other things that have been going on since last school year.

"Really, what could be worse?" you ask.

Trevor tells you, "Last year they put itching powder in his football uniform. After that, they took his helmet, so he couldn't play with the team. The next thing they did was to put things online about Eric, lying about who he really is. They fabricated an arrest record for assault.

"This year, I'm pretty sure the guys have gone into a central computer to change his grades to failing."

"It looks to me like he still has friends," you say.

"Yes, he still has us," Trevor says. "But the worse thing was that we all used to be friends until they turned on him. Since they know Eric so well, they also know how to upset him."

Continue on page 17.

The next thing they did was make sure no one would hang out with him, by posting things online about him lying about who he really is. They fabricated an arrest record for assault."

"It looks to me like he still has friends," you say.

"Yes, he still has us," Trevor says. "But the worse thing was that we all used to be friends until they turned on him. They all know Eric really well."

It's time to choose a path:

If Trevor finds out about the gun—continue on page 15.

If you decide to take the gun home—continue on page 19.

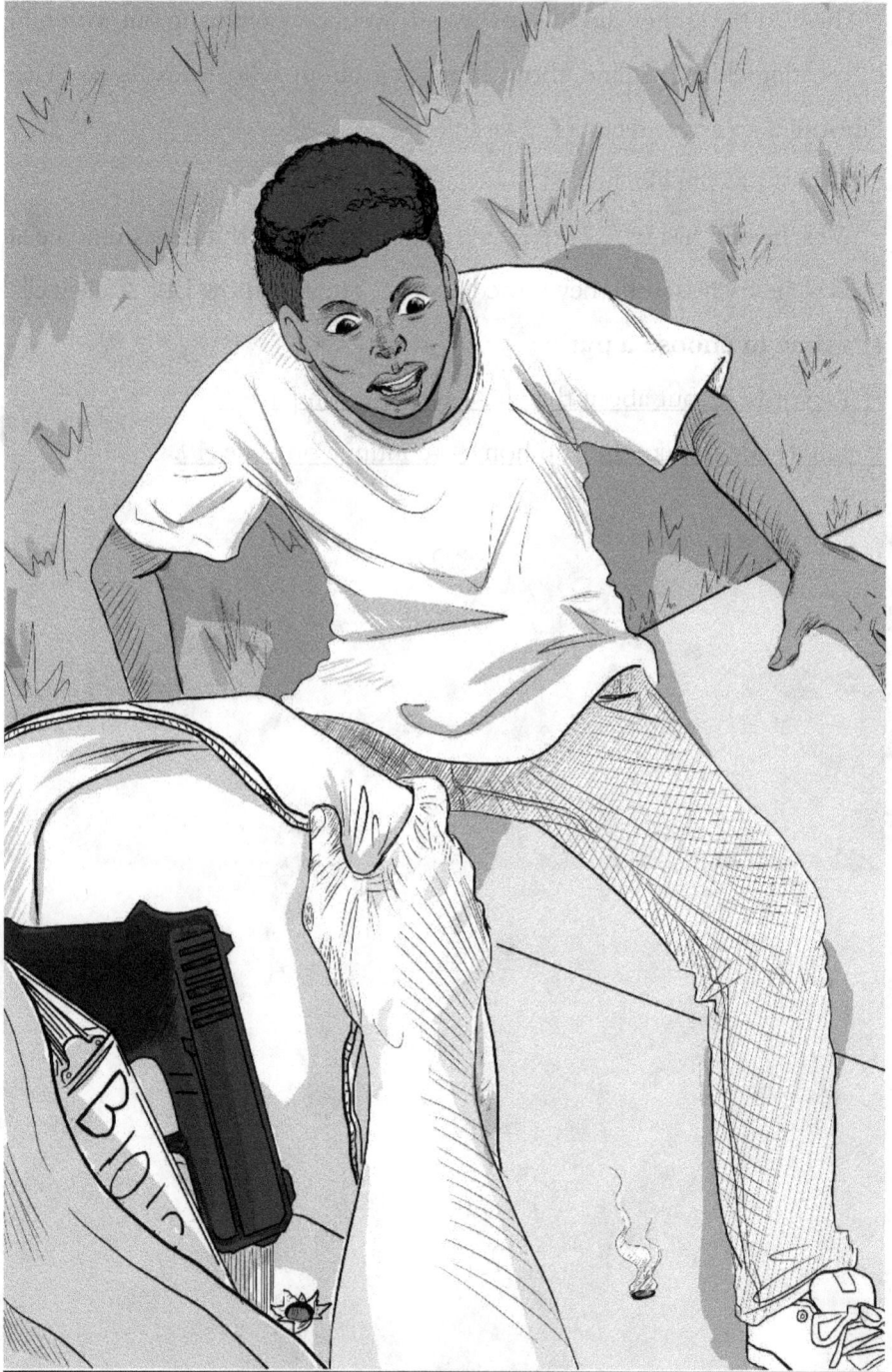

If Trevor finds out about the gun

You decide to tell Trevor about your fear that Eric might hurt someone with the gun. You don't tell him that you have the gun in your backpack, but you ask if he thinks Eric will hurt someone.

Trevor says, "No, I don't think so."

You reach into the backpack to feel for the gun and accidentally shoot a hole through your backpack nearly shooting Trevor in his foot.

"What the. . ." Trevor says. He's scared and his voice is much higher than usual. "You. . . you have a gun? You could've shot me. Where did you get the gun?"

You admit, "I took it, so Eric wouldn't take the gun to school. I was afraid to speak up, since I don't really know anyone."

"What did you plan to do with it?" Trevor asks.

"Uh, well, I don't really know. Probably take it to my parents."

Now Trevor is angry with you. He shouts, "Well, now you can't."

"Why not?"

He continues his tirade, "You shot the gun, and nearly shot me." Now, if you get caught with a gun, you could be charged with a crime." [22]

Continue on page 21.

If Trevor says Eric's a good guy and he wouldn't take the gun to school, you should believe him, but something just doesn't feel right.

You finally fall asleep and wake up to your mom standing over your bed. "You must've overslept," she says. "Now you need to hurry and get dressed."

Just as you're eating breakfast, Trevor comes to pick you up for school.

"I'm good," you say. "I'll meet up with you later."

You start out walking to school alone. Two of your new friends, Lisa and Sara, join you. "Do you really think Eric would take a gun to school?" you ask the two girls.

Lisa answers, nearly spitting out her words "I don't think he will, but I think he should. He's taken enough from those bullies."

Sara answers more calmly than her friend, "I hope and pray that he doesn't. He could hurt someone and then his future would be down the toilet."

You agree with Sara.

Why should you feel bad about other people's bad choices? After all, you don't even really know any of the kids you hung out with yesterday.

Continue on page 18.

Soon you are home again and begin working on homework.

You continue to think about the gun and worry that if you say something, you will lose your chance to have new friends.

What should you do? It's time to choose a path:

If you tell your parents about the gun—continue on page 31.

If you tell Trevor that you have something else to do the next day—continue on page 30.

If you don't say anything, because you're curious and want to see the gun again—continue on page 27.

When you enter your school, everything seems noisy, chaotic and normal. There are no police officers hanging around. The first bell rings and all the kids in the hallway scramble toward their classrooms.

You still have a sneaking feeling that things aren't right. That feeling won't go away. After first period, you go into the bathroom and throw up. Then you go to the office and ask to go home.

What should you do? It's time to choose a path:

If you believe Trevor—but something just doesn't feel right—continue on page 20.

If you decide to tell the counselor about Eric being bullied—continue on page 42

If Eric takes the gun to school—continue on page 81.

If you take the gun home

You continue home with the gun in your backpack.

At home, you try to get up the courage to tell your parents about the gun. Your hands are sweating. You are anxious and filled with fear. You had never handled a gun before today, and now you've stolen a weapon and it's sitting in your backpack. You really aren't sure, but you think the gun is still loaded.

You tell your parents the whole story about the bullies bothering Eric. "Eric showed a gun to the group at his house, and each of us handled the loaded gun."

"You didn't!" your mom exclaims.

With alarm in his voice, Dad says, "That's very dangerous. What if someone got hurt?"

You continue. "Someone suggested that Eric should take the gun to school to deal with bullies."

Your mom's eyes open wide. She throws her hands in the air and says, "Oh no!"

Your dad's expression turns dark and angry. He says, "I hope you did something!"

"Yes, I did. Mom, Dad, wait here a minute," you tell them.

You then go get your backpack. "I took the gun from Eric's house because I was afraid Eric would take the weapon to school and shoot someone."

"What? You stole a gun?" your mom asks. "You're carrying a loaded gun in your backpack?"

She collapses into a nearby chair, nearly fainting.

Continue on page 25.

It is possible that Eric has brought the gun to school. You're sure there are better ways to solve bullying problems.

Are you the one who can make a difference, or are you too new and too chicken to do anything? After all, no one told you to watch Eric's back.

You change your mind about going home and head toward your next class. You're feeling so nervous that your heart seems to be pounding in your ears. This is only the second day of school and there's no way you want to mess things up.

Trevor and Sara come up to you in the hall. With panic in his voice, Trevor says, "Eric doesn't look well. We all need to talk to him. I saw one of the bullies trip him in the hall. I'm afraid that he's going to get revenge. Since no one knows about the bullying, it could all be blamed on Eric."

Sara says, "I'm going with you to talk to him."

You agree to go with Trevor as well. Trevor takes you and Sara to Eric's classroom. Before the bell rings at the start of class, he grabs Eric by the arm and says, "We need to talk."

Eric comes out into the hallway and seems shaken up. He asks, "What's wrong?"

Continue on page 23.

You and Trevor come up with a plan to put the gun back.

"We'll both walk back to Eric's house and I'll ring the back doorbell," Trevor says.

"When Eric comes to the door, you keep him busy while I go in through the front door and put the gun back," you finish.

Everything goes according to your plan. After putting the gun back upstairs, you go out the front door and come around the back of Eric's house to hang out with the guys.

"Eric," you ask, "Were you really planning to take the gun to school?"

"Uh, no. I don't think so."

"Well, you can't," Trevor says, with warning in his voice. "Something really bad will happen. You could accidentally shoot someone, and you'll get arrested. That will really mess up your future."

Continue on page 24.

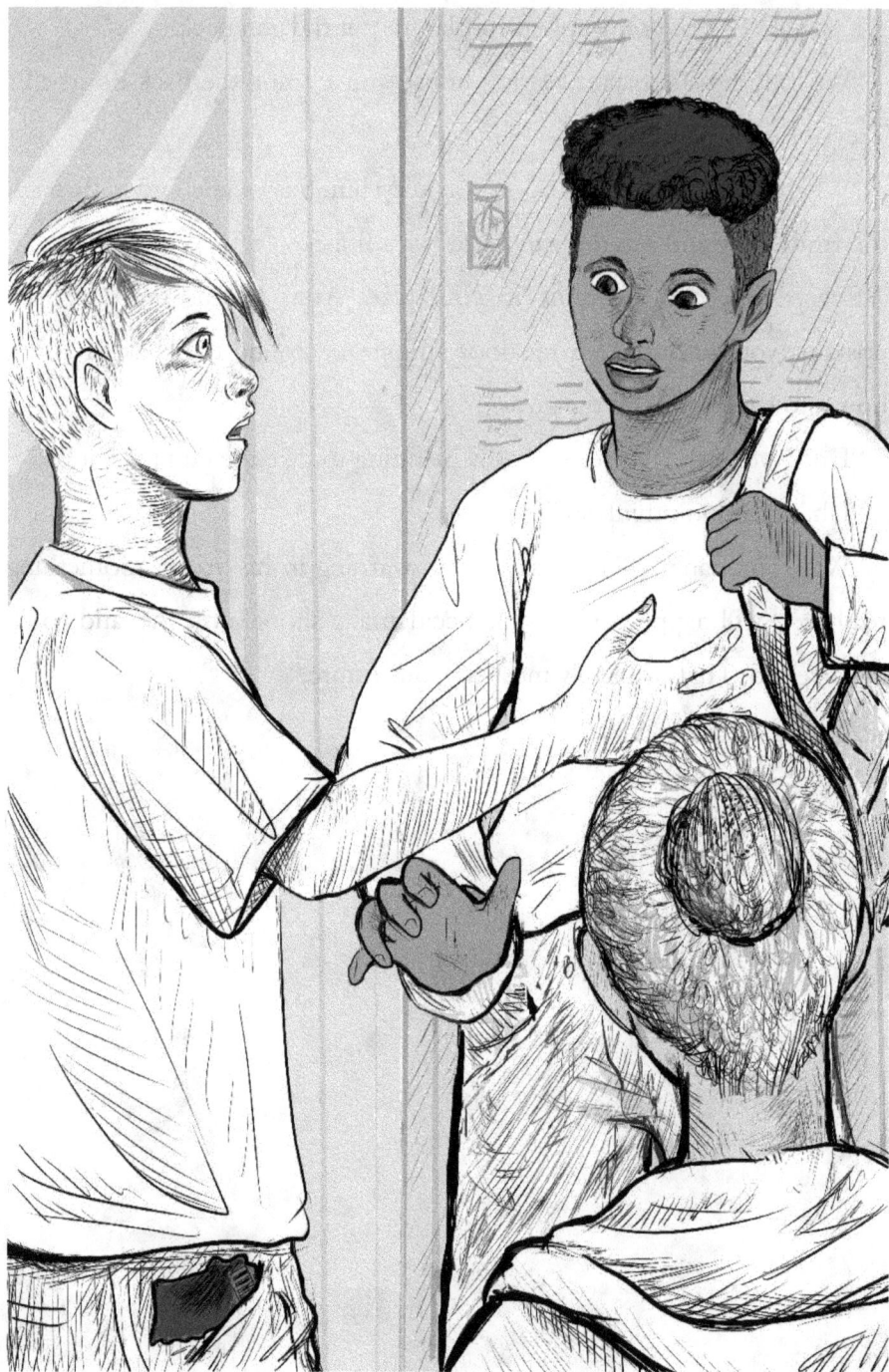

"You tell me," Trevor says. "You seem very shaken up and we're worried that you aren't okay."

"I, I am. Y-y-y-yes I'm okay," Eric says. "I have it all figured out. I'm really going to get those guys this time. I'm not going to let them keep bullying me. I'm tired of being the victim."

"What do you mean, Eric?" Trevor asks.

A big smile comes to Eric's face. "I have the gun and I'm going to show them who's boss." You turn pale when he shows the gun he has in his pocket. All of you back up a step.

"No, Eric!" you say. "No, you can't do that."

None of the kids seem to notice the gym teacher coming down the hall behind you.

"Eric, I need to use your phone for a minute," Trevor says. Eric hands him the phone and Trevor has you text Eric's father. "Tell him there's a problem at school."

You take Eric's phone and find his dad's number. You text him: *This is a friend of Eric's. There's a bullying situation at school. Eric is in serious trouble and needs you right away! SOS!*

Continue on page 32

"Yeah, sure," Eric says. "But what about protection? I'm sick of being bullied and just want to make it stop."

You suggest that the whole group go with Eric to talk to his parents and the principal.

Eric agrees and the three of you set up a plan.

You realize that by taking the gun in your backpack, you put both yourself and Trevor in danger. [*22] The gun went off, nearly shooting Trevor in the foot. That was a very close call! No one got shot, you didn't have to explain to your parents about the gun, and Eric will get help with his bullying problem. This came out better than expected.

The End

Your mom continues, "What did you intend to do with the gun? Were *you* planning to take it to school? Were you going to sneak back into Eric's house and put the gun back?"

"No, Mom! Well, I don't know. I just wanted to protect the other kids at school. I didn't think about what I'd do with the gun."

Your dad walks with you over to Trevor's house to talk to his parents about the gun. Trevor and his dad go with you and your dad back to Eric's house.

"It's your responsibility to explain to Eric's dad what happened today and why you have the gun," your dad says.

When you get to Eric's house, his dad comes to the door. When he sees all of you standing there, he hollers for Eric. They invite you in. You all sit down. Your dad nudges you. You explain, "Eric showed us a gun today."

His dad gives him a stern look and gets to his feet.

"What! You kids were playing around with a loaded gun!"

Eric nods his head.

Continue on page 26.

You continue, "I've never seen a real gun before. When the other kids held the weapon, someone told Eric to take the gun to school, so he could deal with the bullies. I took this gun home because I thought someone would be shot and I just wanted to protect Eric and the other kids at school. I know I was wrong, but I don't know anyone very well and I guess I didn't have the courage to speak up."

Eric's dad turns to him, speaking more quietly now, "Son, did you plan to take the gun to school?"

"Well, we were talking about it. I'm not sure. It's been on my mind a lot lately." Eric starts to cry and says, "Dad, the kids on the football team won't leave me alone. I did think about showing them the gun, just to get their attention. I don't think I would've actually shot anyone."

Eric's dad also has tears in his eyes. He says to you, "Thank you for trying to keep everyone safe, but that's not your job! Did you even think that it was unsafe to have a loaded gun in your backpack?"

"Yes, I did start thinking about that, and that's when I told my parents," you say. Realizing the seriousness of the situation, tears come to your eyes, as well.

Continue on page 28.

You try to do your homework, but your mind keeps returning to thoughts about the gun. You wonder what it would feel like to shoot a gun. You wonder if Eric will show it to you again. You remember that Eric said the gun was loaded. What's the worst that could happen?

You don't have to wonder for long because the next day after school, Eric and Trevor invite you to hang out again. You thought for sure one of your friends would've reported the gun, but you knew it couldn't be you. You are new at the school and wouldn't dare start out by tattling on your new friends. Besides, you really want a chance to shoot the gun. That would be so cool!

What should you do? It's time to choose a path:

If you choose Target Practice—continue on page 43

If you choose Six Kids, One Gun—continue on page 44.

If you choose Hide and Seek—continue on page 56.

Your dad says, "It's much better to tell someone before things get to this point. None of you kids should have even touched a loaded gun without supervision. What if you got hurt, or hurt someone else by taking the gun?"

You and everyone else agree.

"I'm so glad no one got hurt," Eric's dad says. "It's my job to protect everyone in this house. Having a loaded gun within the reach of kids like you, isn't safe. I'm so sorry this happened. I'm responsible and I can tell you, that gun is going to be disarmed and put into a gun safe with all the other guns in this house."

Eric's dad disarms the gun in front of all of you. He sets the gun on his table. He then shakes hands with you, your dad, Trevor and his dad. "Thanks to you, everyone is much safer around here. Eric and I will go talk to the principal the first thing in the morning and settle this bullying problem once and for all."

Everyone says "goodnight," and you, your dad and neighbors go home.

You realize that you handled this situation wrong.

Continue on page 29.

You could have been hurt or you could have hurt someone else. You never should've handled the loaded gun in the first place but taking it home in your backpack was very dangerous and should've never happened. Even though this was the wrong way to handle a dangerous situation, it still turned out much better than expected.

The next day, Eric's dad invites your group to come back to his house. A police officer is also invited over to talk to all of you. He tells the group about the dangers of handling a loaded gun and the consequences of taking a gun to school. The officer makes it clear that if Eric had taken the gun to school, he could've been charged with illegal possession of a firearm on school property, and possibly charged with illegal discharge of a firearm. Even though he's a teenager, he can be charged in adult court and serve time in prison. If Eric shot someone at school, he may possibly be sentenced to serve life in prison. [1, 23]

*See picture on page 35

The End

<u>If you tell Trevor that you have something else to do the next day:</u>

You don't tell your parents about the gun, but you can't stop thinking about how someone could get shot. Rather than dealing with such an uncomfortable situation and knowing that Eric and the group will take the gun out for target practice the next day, you decide to avoid the group after school. On your second day of school, once again, Trevor is there to show you around to your classes. You have lunch together with the same group. During lunch break, you go into the hallway and call your mom to pick you up from school. You don't want to take any chances of being talked into going home with Eric, not with a loaded, unlocked gun in the house.

After school, you tell Trevor, "Hey, will you let the group know I'm not going to Eric's after school?"

Trevor says, "Oh, I'm sorry you can't make it."

When your mom comes, she takes you to the mall to get some school supplies. You go home and work on a school project but keep watching out your window to see if Trevor is coming home.

<u>Continue on page 38.</u>

If you tell your parents about the gun

Your mom comes into your room and asks about your first day at the new school.

"Well, Trevor showed me around the school. At lunchtime we ate with a group of his friends, then after school Trevor took me over to his friend Eric's house with the same a group of kids I met at lunchtime.

"Were parents' home at Eric's house?" asks your mom.

"No, his parents weren't there. At first, we went outside and played football, then came in for snacks, but. . ." you hesitate.

"What? What is it?"

"Well, it didn't seem so bad at first, but I can't stop thinking about it, so it must be bad," you say.

"You weren't drinking, were you?" asks your mom.

"No, Mom. Eric took us upstairs and showed us a gun. It was loaded and in his mom's nightstand. Eric took out the gun and pretended to shoot at things around the room making the sound of shooting, 'Pow, pow, pow.'"

Your mom's mouth drops open. "Oh, no! A loaded gun?"

Continue on page 34.

"You need to go home now!" Trevor says. "You've messed up, big time. You can't bring a gun to school. Someone will get hurt. You cannot do this!"

The teacher hears all the commotion. When he hears the word "gun," he also notices that Eric has a gun in his pocket. You see the teacher as he comes closer while talking on his radio. "Security, we have a gun situation. I repeat, we have a gun on school property, hallway #2." Eric seems alarmed and looks like he might run.

"You kids need to slowly back away from Eric and head to the nearest classroom. The security officer is on his way."

As you inch away, you hear the teacher talking to Eric.

"Eric, son, this is a serious crime. You have a gun on school property, and I heard you say you want to harm someone. Do you really want to shoot someone?"

You look back at Eric.

He shrugs. "The guys on the football team have been bullying me since last year and I can't take it anymore."

That scares you. Here he is with a gun and even after he gets caught, he's still not sure if he wants to hurt someone.

The principal speaks over the intercom. "We have a lockdown situation. No one leaves or enters this building. If you are in the hallway, quickly enter the nearest classroom. I repeat, no one leaves this building. This is a lockdown situation."

Two security officers come to the scene. Eric hands over the gun and he is immediately taken into custody.

Continue on page 33

Kids in the school are panicking, trying to get out of the hallway. You, Sara and Trevor hurry to the nearest classroom. You find yourself in a cooking class. The teacher locks the door.

You're filled with both fear and relief. Fear because you can see how upset Eric is and that he wants revenge. Relief that three of you saw that something was wrong and stopped Eric in time. You also seriously hope that Eric will get help.

Everyone in the classroom, where you are waiting, runs to the window. You see several police cars arrive and officers surround the building. Trevor tells you that Eric's dad has arrived and points to a man talking to the principal outside. Soon after, Eric is taken out in handcuffs. Everyone in the room gasps.

"It's Eric! What did he do?" someone asks.

Some girls are crying. Kids are wondering what happened. Someone says, "I think we had a school shooting!"

Someone else says, "I didn't hear any gunshots."

You, Trevor and Sara let everyone know that they are safe. Trevor says, "We saw the security officer take the gun. The school security and the police have it under control."

After an hour, the classroom doors are unlocked. The news has reported a school shooter and parents panic and pick up their kids early. Nothing about school feels normal now. You wonder if it will ever feel safe or normal again.

Continue on page 41

"Yes, and Mom, each of us had a turn holding the gun. One of the kids told Eric to take the gun to school tomorrow to show the bullies who's boss. I'm really worried what will happen. I'm also scared that by telling, I won't have any friends at my new school. Trevor is good friends with Eric and he . . . he might turn on me too."

Mom says, "I never imagined having to deal with a situation like this. It is very new to me. Sometimes we have to make hard choices, but this shouldn't be a hard choice. What do you think you should do?"

"I think someone should stop Eric before anybody gets hurt. I just met the kids but maybe I can save someone's life, even if they don't like me after today.

"We need to tell someone, Mom."

"Yes, of course you're right," your mom says. "I knew you'd come up with the answer. We don't know anyone else around here, so I think we should go talk to Trevor's parents."

You nod your head and you both walk next door.

When Trevor answers the door, your mom says, "Trevor, will you please go get your parents? We all need to talk."

Continue on page 36.

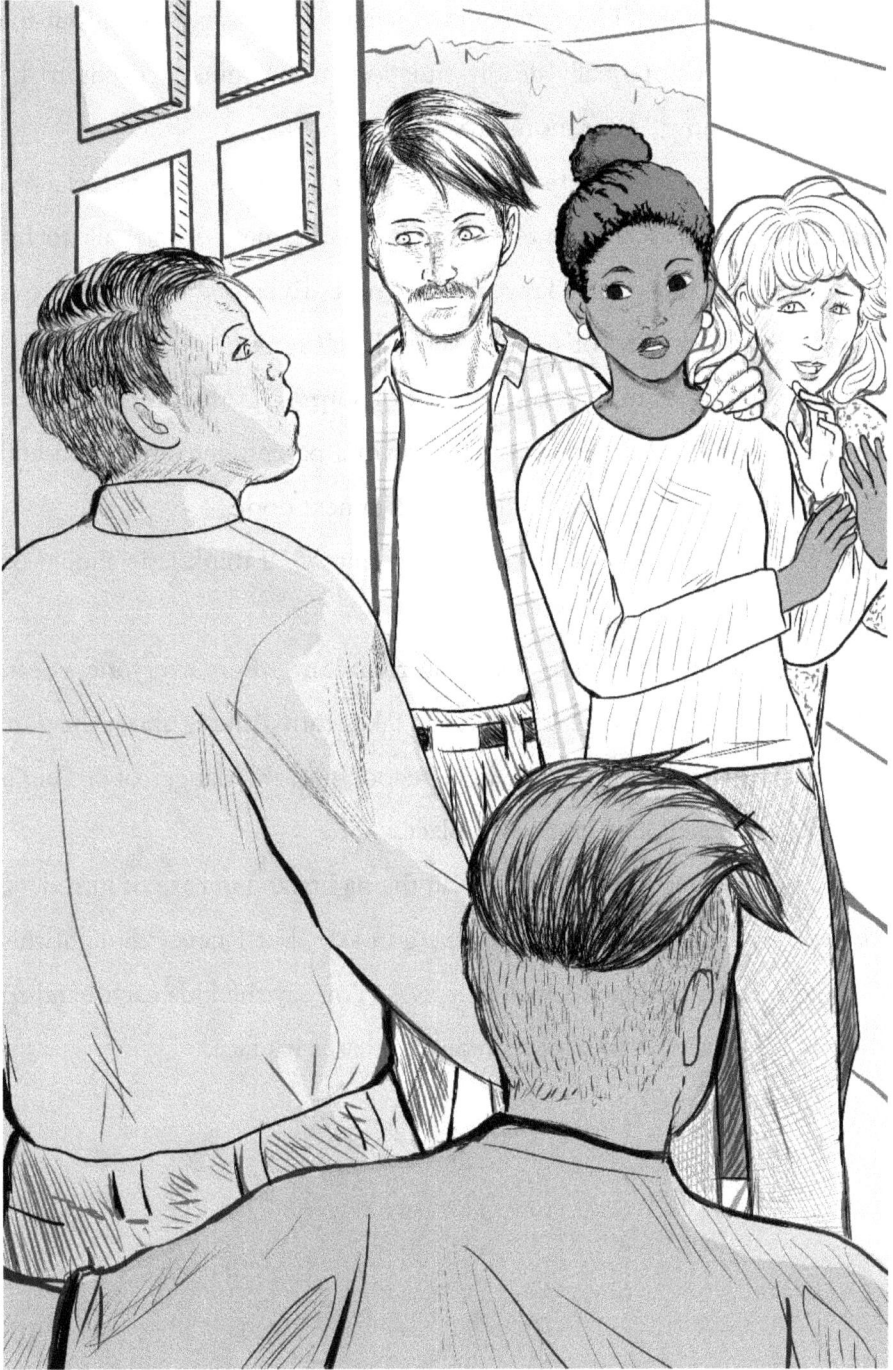

You, your mom and Trevor take turns telling Trevor's parents about the gun. "This is a potentially deadly situation, and I think it needs to be handled right now," your mom says.

Trevor's parents agree. His mom is wringing her hands. His dad tells you that they know Eric's parents very well. "We all need to go talk to his parents about the gun," Trevor's dad says. Everyone gets into your neighbor's car and Trevor's dad drives to Eric's house.

Eric's dad comes to the door. A look of surprise crosses his face when he sees all of you standing outside. Trevor's parents introduce you and your mom as the new family who moved in next door.

"We need to talk," Trevor's dad says sternly. "I think Eric should be in on this conversation."

He invites all of you into his living room and offers everyone a seat. After he returns with Eric, each person takes turns talking about the gun, the worry that Eric might take it to school, and the danger of having a loaded gun around kids in the first place.

Eric's dad admits they have a gun in the nightstand in case of intruders. "I also have other guns locked in the gun safe, but I never thought this gun would be a problem. Obviously, it is. You say the kids each handled the gun?" He asks. A look of incredulity crosses his face.

Continue on page 37.

Yes," you and Trevor answer.

"Eric, were you thinking of taking the gun to school?" his dad asks.

"Uh, well, I have been bullied at school ever since last year. Someone suggested I should take the gun to school to show the bullies who's boss. After they all left, I thought about taking it to school. I even put the gun into my backpack. Then I put it back upstairs. Now, I have the gun in my backpack again."

"Son give me the gun! Go get your backpack. I'm locking this gun in the safe. I don't want any of these kids and their parents feeling unsafe in our home or at school."

Eric leaves the room and comes back with his backpack and hands the gun to his dad. His dad removes the clip of bullets and sets the gun on the table beside him.

Continue on page 40.

You hope that things go well at Eric's house but rather than risking the new friendship, you avoid the situation all together.

You sit by the window for quite a while, before you see Trevor running down the street in a panic. He enters his house and watches out the window, peeking through the curtain. Maybe he thinks no one will know he's home, but you can see him peeking out. You wonder what's going on. Did something happen to spook him? At least, you know he's home.

You get up the courage to go over and talk to Trevor. You ring the doorbell but for a while, no one answers. "I know you're there, Trevor. I saw you go inside."

Trevor comes to the door and stands mostly behind the entrance, peeking out. "What do you want?"

You ask, "Trevor, did something happen? Are you okay?"

"No, no I'm not okay." He seems to be checking his arms, legs, then his torso. He opens the door wider as he checks his face in a mirror by the door.

"Okay. I'm alright. You can come in. Wait, you didn't bring anyone with you, did you?"

Continue on page 39.

"No. Who would I bring with me?"

"The. . . the cops. You didn't bring the cops, did you?"

"No, why would I bring the cops? What's wrong?"

"The gun. Eric had the gun. He shot someone. He might have shot everyone. I don't know. Loud shots went off. Blood, in his house. Blood everywhere. I don't know who was shot. Maybe Eric. Maybe his dad, and a girl. Lisa was shot too. Sara, Tyler and I ran home and never looked back.

The cops might think I did it. I'm not going back. I can't. Can't return. Won't go! No, I won't. I didn't do it. I would never do it. You should go now! You need to go."

"No," you say. "I didn't go back to Eric's house. I went home. You shouldn't have gone either. Why did you go?"

"I, I wanted to shoot the gun. It was scary and exciting to hold a loaded gun. I wanted to shoot at a target, but then everything went wrong. Sara slipped on the step. Eric had his finger on the trigger. He was pretending to shoot at different things around the house, like he did yesterday. Suddenly, Sara bumped into Eric and he accidentally shot Lisa. She fell. Continue on page 47.

"Taking a gun to school will create much bigger problems!" Eric's dad exclaims. "Eric, I feel bad that you're feeling threatened at school. You should've come to us about the bullying. We can meet with your coach and the principal and make sure it doesn't happen again. We'll take care of this first thing tomorrow," his dad says.

If Eric had taken a gun to school, he could've been charged as an adult. There are very strict laws about having weapons on school property. Even though Eric was bullied at school, bringing a gun to school wouldn't have solved anything, in fact, it would've ruined Eric's future. [*9]

You're glad you spoke up about the gun. Eric already had the gun in his backpack and was planning to take it to school the next day. What would've happened if you hadn't told your mom?

What a relief!

The End

After school, you tell your parents about Eric, the gun you saw at his house the day before, and about Eric bringing the gun to school.

Your mom is horrified and reluctant to let you out of her sight. Your new friends want to gather at Trevor's house. But, before allowing you to go next door, your mom checks with his parents to make sure they don't have any unlocked guns in the house. She also says you are never allowed into a house where there are no parents at home. All the kids are sad and worried about Eric. What will happen to him now? You are pretty sure Eric will never be back at school.

The next day, police officers and counselors come to talk to your school's student body. An officer begins by saying, "As you may already know, Eric was caught with a gun at school yesterday. He has been arrested and taken to a detention center. He could be charged with possession of a weapon on school property. Also, because he wanted to harm someone, he could be in the custody of juvenile detention until he is twenty-one years old, or be charged as an adult, even though he's still a teenager."

Next you hear from a counselor, who says, "with the gun in police custody and Eric in detention, everyone is safe. No minors will ever see or touch that gun again. At the end of this assembly, anyone who is afraid or concerned will be given an opportunity to speak with a counselor." [15, 25]

You later find out that Eric's dad could also be charged for contributing to the delinquency of a minor, as well as a weapons charge for allowing a minor easy access to a loaded weapon. [17]

The End

If you decide to tell the counselor about Eric being bullied:

While you're in the office, you change your mind and ask to talk to a counselor. In your mind, you wonder how you can talk about Eric without getting him into trouble. But while waiting, you still feel the need to talk to a counselor about Eric. Maybe your new group of friends will excuse you for telling. If not, you'll need to find new friends after today. When you get in to see the counselor, you introduce yourself, and then say, "I'm new in this school."

The counselor asks, "How are you getting along?" Have you made new friends here?"

"Yes, I like it here so far. I have a new group of friends, but that's what I want to talk to you about. I heard that Eric is being bullied and he hasn't asked for help."

"Do you know Eric's last name?" she asks.

"No, I don't," you say. "But he's good friends with Trevor and he was on the football team last year."

She looks up the football team from last year and says, "I found him here. It's Eric Brown."

You ask the counselor to talk to Eric because you want him to get help and you're worried that he may feel desperate enough to hurt someone. Continue on page 49.

If you choose Target Practice

The day before, Eric mentioned that he would take the group outside for target practice. You've thought of nothing else since you first held the gun in your hand yesterday. You continued to think about it last night, during school today and on your way to Eric's house. You're very anxious and can hardly wait for your turn to shoot the gun.

You walk with Trevor over to Eric's house. Eric meets your group outside the door of his house. You notice that the others have already arrived. Eric leads all of you around the outside of his house to his back yard for target practice.

Eric tells the group, "I have cans, bottles and three targets set up in the backyard."

You see large paper targets with black silhouettes, in the shape of a person set up on three separate, close together trees, each one with points for shooting certain parts of the stranger's body. Shooting the middle of the paper silhouette will give you ten points and shooting him in the head will also give you ten points.

Continue on page 77.

<u>Six Kids, One Gun</u>

This time the group of six enters the house and there's no small talk. You all head up to Eric's parent's room and he takes out the gun. He removes the clip and demonstrates how to load the gun by placing the clip back into the firearm.

"We have sixteen bullets and an extra clip. Let's go outside so we can all have a chance to shoot this thing," he says.

You each head down the stairs with Eric in the lead, holding up the gun.

Once again, Eric pretends to shoot with his finger on the trigger. Sara, the girl behind him stops short and bumps into Eric. With his finger already on the trigger, the gun goes off with a loud popping sound, shooting Lisa, who is now one step ahead of him. She's hit in the shoulder. The impact pushes her into the wall. She stumbles on the stairs and can't stop herself from falling.

Eric is shaken! He looks at the gun, then at Lisa in disbelief.

<u>Continue on page 46.</u>

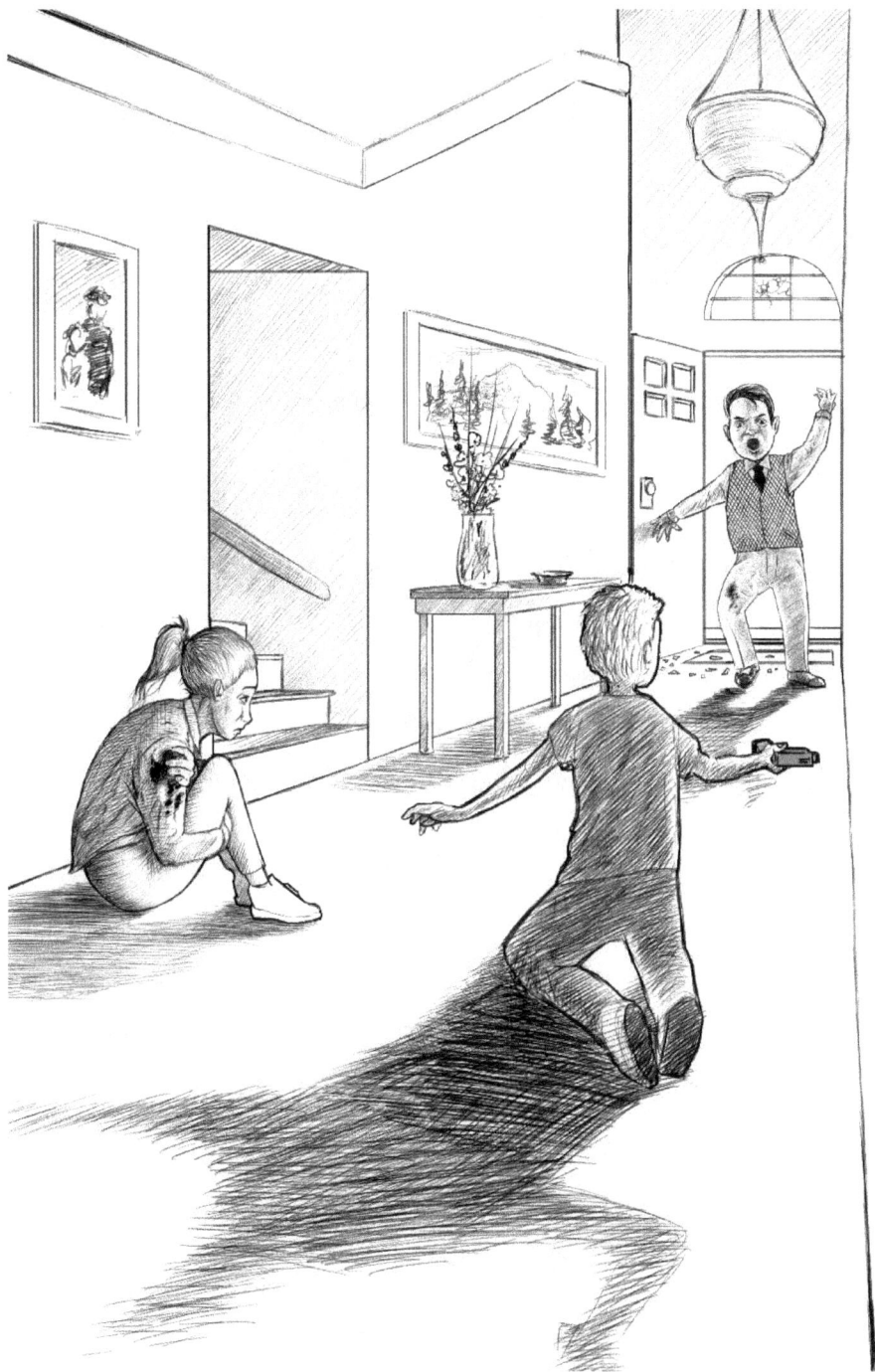

Lisa isn't aware that she's been shot until she touches her shoulder and gets blood on her fingers.

"I felt something hot, and for a moment I thought I was burned," she says, after landing on her knees at the bottom of the steps. She holds up her hand, covered in her own blood. "I think I've been shot!"

You all gasp. Blood seems to be everywhere. Lisa leans against a dining room chair and sobs. Eric goes down the steps to check on Lisa. He's still holding the gun when his dad opens the front door and sees his son, holding a gun.

"Eric, what are *you* doing?" his dad says in a sharp voice.

Eric turns toward his dad. He is so alarmed that he shoots the gun again. The loud sound of the gun shooting, along with the blood and smell of gun powder seem overwhelming. The next bullet hits Eric's dad in the leg. He stumbles a few steps forward, trying to get to Lisa. Eric's dad collapses onto his hurt side, yelling out in pain. Both injured people lay on the floor, bleeding from their gunshot wounds.[*3]

Continue on page 51.

JILL AMMON VANDERWOOD

His dad came into the house and said, "'Eric, what are *you* doing?'" Eric turned around and accidentally shot his dad. Then another bullet hit the window before Eric dropped the gun. There's blood everywhere. I grabbed Sara and we ran out of there. We didn't want to get shot or blamed for the shooting."

"Trevor, you need to go back. You won't be blamed. The police can test your hands for gun powder. If you didn't shoot the gun, it won't show up on your hands."

"Are you sure," Trevor asks.

"Yes, I'm sure. Also, you said that Eric dropped the gun, so he's not going to shoot you. We need to call 911 so the people who are shot can get help. Then we need to go back and stay there until help arrives."

Trevor still refuses to make the call. You alone can't convince him.

You go home and talk to your mom about the shooting.

Continue on page 62.

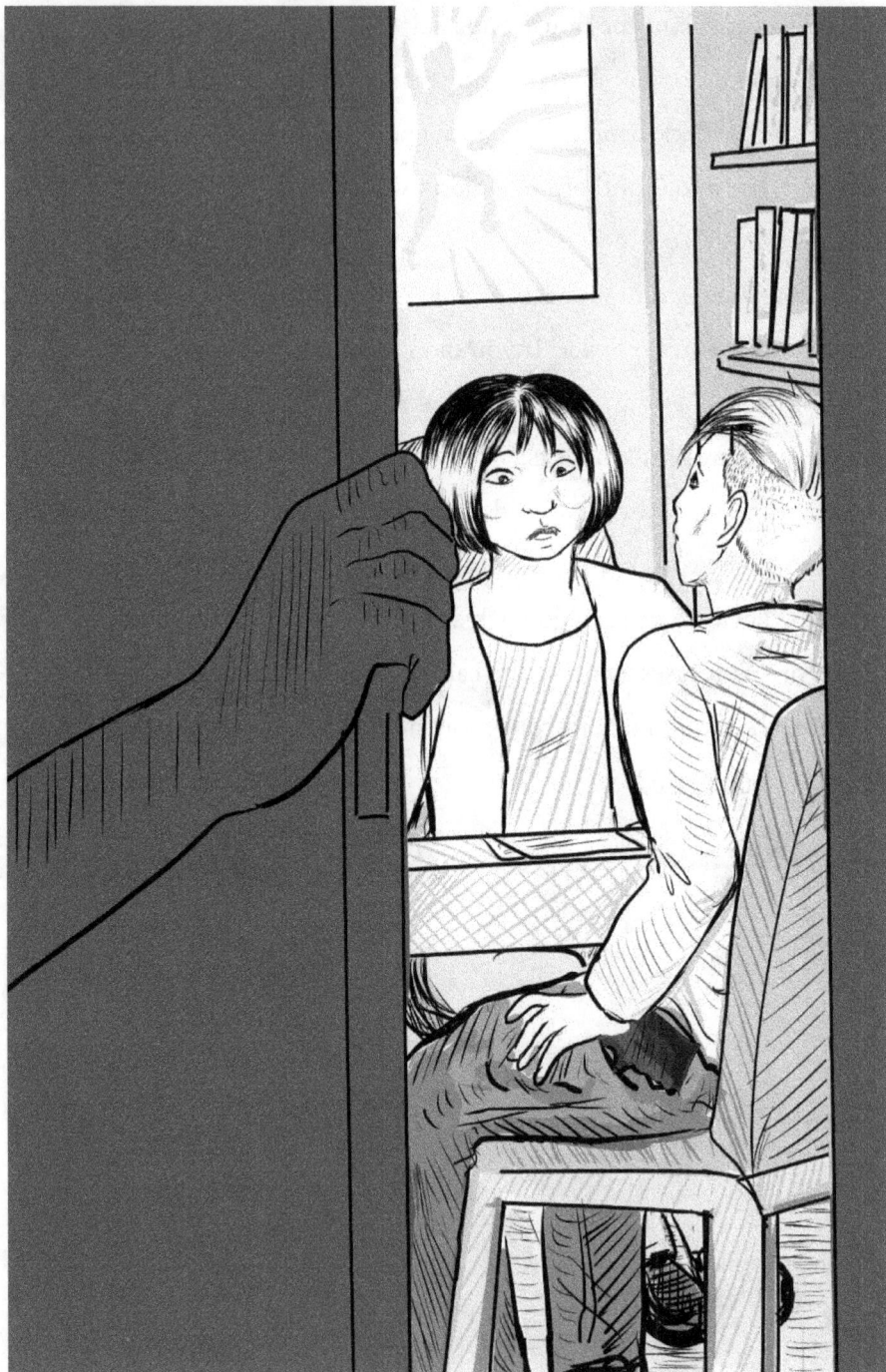

The counselor asks you, "Did Eric tell you he wants to hurt someone?"

You say, "No, but some of his friends told him he should get them back and I'm worried that if he does, he'll be in bigger trouble than the kids picking on him."

The counselor thanks you. She says she won't tell him about the conversation and excuses you. As you're leaving, she calls Eric into the office.

When he arrives, Eric walks right past but doesn't notice you. You watch and listen through the crack in the door, where it isn't quite shut. You see that he's sweating and seems agitated.

"Eric, it was pointed out to me that you're being bullied. Is that correct?" the counselor asks.

At first, Eric tries to deny the bullying, but he finally admits that, "Yes, I'm being bullied."

"Eric, it's not bad to admit things aren't going well at school and that it's really making you angry. What kind of things are going on?"

He adjusts himself in his seat and begins telling the counselor about the kind of bullying that's been going on. He tells about his grades being changed.

Continue on page 50.

She says she heard about that, "I can send a note to all of your teachers asking for your final grades, then compare those grades with the ones in our computer system."

Eric nods his head. Then he tells her about the internet post with him being arrested for assault and robbery. "But that never even happened," he says. "They wanted me off the team just because I wouldn't go along with their weekend drinking parties. That doesn't mean I'm a felon."

"I see," the counselor says. "A friend of yours is concerned that your anger for the bullies could turn into an act of revenge."

Eric is wearing a long baggy shirt. You notice that he has something in his pocket that he keeps running his fingers over and wonder if he did bring the gun to school. "I really don't want to hurt anyone," he says. "I just want the bullies to stop!" He stands up.

"I really need help to make this stop, before I do something I might regret." He then sits back down.

Continue on page 55.

Eric is so startled, he shoots another bullet. *Bang!* This time hitting the front window which shatters into a million pieces.

You and the three kids are stunned. You aren't shot, but you're not sure if Eric has been shot. There is so much blood. Dark, red blood everywhere.

Your neighbor, Trevor, shouts, "Run! Get out of here. Now!" Trevor, Tyler and Sara step around the bodies and run out the front door as fast as they can. Sara tries to stop and check on her friend, but Trevor pulls her away and out the door.

What should you do? It's time to choose a path:

If you call 911 and wait for the police—continue on page 54.

If you panic and leave with Trevor—continue on page 52.

If you panic and leave with Trevor

Panic comes over all of you. You follow Trevor and get out of there. You can't seem to think for yourself. Trevor is your friend and he says we should leave, so you follow him out the door.

You know you shouldn't be playing with a gun. You knew it was dangerous and that someone could get hurt. And now they have. You could've stopped it by telling someone the day before, but you were scared. You wanted a chance to have a new group of friends, but now look what happened, because you didn't say anything. You are becoming a follower. You could be better than that. Someone is hurt and here you are running, out of fear and panic. You could go back. You should go back.

No, they might think you did this. You didn't do this! You didn't cause this. You don't own a gun and you didn't shoot anyone.

What should you do? It's not too late to choose a new path:

If you try to go back on your own—continue on page 59.

If you go home and don't tell anyone what happened for about an hour—continue on page 57.

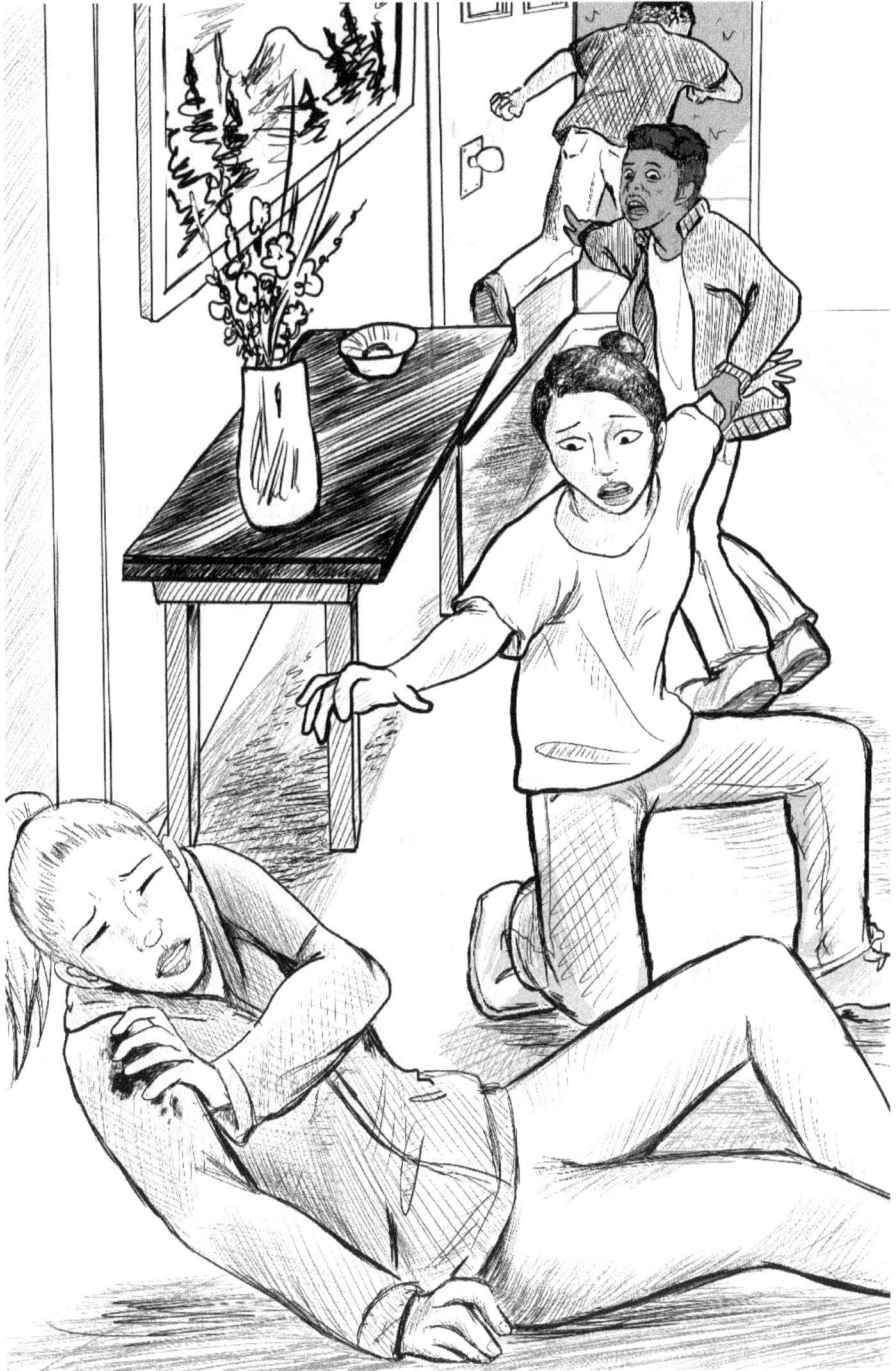

If you call 911 and wait for the police

You stay at Eric's house and check on those who've been shot. You take out your cell phone and dial 911. The dispatcher answers: "911 what is your emergency?"

You try your best to explain the situation. "Gun, someone has a gun. Someone got shot! Hurry!"

"Slow down, take a breath and start over," the 911 operator says. "How many people are in the house?"

You remember that there were six kids, including you, but some of them left. Then you count, outload. "Eric, his dad, Lisa and me. There are four people in the house now."

The operator asks, "Are you hurt?"

You quickly check yourself, "No, I'm not hurt."

"Is everyone else hurt?" You look at Eric's dad and Lisa, collapsed on the floor. Eric's walking around with blood on his hands. There's blood on the floor and the wall. Eric doesn't seem to be hurt. He's just covered with other people's blood

"Well, I think two people are hurt. I can't tell with all the blood in the house," you say.

"Do you know your location?" she asks.

Continue on page 66

The counselor says, "Cyberbullying is illegal in this state, also, changing someone's grades is subject to termination from this school. We'll get someone right on it. No one has the right to make you feel unsafe in your own school."

You continue to watch Eric through the crack in the door. Once again, Eric fingers the object in his pocket.

The counselor hands Eric a piece of paper. "I want you to write down the names of the boys who're picking on you."

At first, Eric pushes the paper away. "No, no I can't."

"Eric is there someone you want to protect?" the counselor asks.

"Uh, well no," he says.

"The only way I can help you and make this go away is for you to give me the names."

Eric takes the piece of paper and writes down the names.

"Okay. That'll help get this taken care of. I can see how upset you are about this. I think I should send you home for the rest of the day.

Continue on page 72.

If you choose Hide and Seek:

The following day, the group of kids arrive at Eric's house after school. Eric grabs the gun and sets up two groups to play hide and seek in his backyard. You're on a team with Sara and Trevor.

Eric counts to fifty while each of you go and hide. First, he finds Lisa hiding in a large empty barrel used to collect rainwater. He goes "Pow! Pow! Pow!" With his mouth and then '*bang*!' He shoots the gun into the air.

Next Eric finds one of the boys—Tyler. He's hiding in a chicken coop. He says, "Pow!" and '*Bang!*' Eric shoots off the gun once more. You know that two have been found.

Eric walks close to where you're hiding in the garage, and says, "I know you're here. Why don't you just come out and get it over with?" But he doesn't see you. He then finds Trevor hiding in the large, child's swimming pool. "Pow!" Then '*bang*' he shoots the gun into the air. Dogs are barking around the neighborhood, but you distinctly hear a '*yelp*!'

Continue on page 83.

If you go home and don't tell anyone what happened for about an hour

You continue toward home and watch Trevor enter his house. "Mom, I'm home!" you yell on your way upstairs to your room.

"How was your first day at school?" your mom asks from the bottom of the steps.

"It was good. Trevor showed me around the school and I met some new kids," you say.

"That's great!" Mom says.

You go to your room and turn on music with your headphones, trying to drown out your conscience. Part of you thinks you should go back to Eric's house. The other part is afraid that things will turn ugly and you and Trevor will be blamed for taking off like that. What kind of person are you? Are you one who abandons others when they need you?

You continue to think, I don't know where Eric lives. But why can't Eric call the police? He's the one who shot the gun. It's not my gun. It wasn't my house. I didn't even shoot the gun.

Continue on page 58.

Why was I there in the first place? I already knew Eric had the gun. I also knew that he planned to take all the kids outside to shoot at a target. All that blood! And the hurt people.

What should I do? Why do I need to do anything?

Because you, Trevor and the other kids left after the shooting, those who were shot could bleed out and no one would know to save them, unless Eric's mom comes home.

You don't tell anyone for about an hour, then your conscience gets the better of you.

You go downstairs and talk to your mom. You tell her all about the gun and what happened. She takes you next door to talk to Trevor's mom. Trevor's mother knows Eric's parents very well. She gets on the phone and calls his mother to tell her what happened.

When Eric's mom answers, Trevor's mom puts the phone on speaker and asks, "I just found out what happened at your house. Are you home?"

You, Trevor and your mom listen in. "I got home about an hour ago. Apparently, Eric was wandering down the street, covered with blood and someone called 911.

Continue on page 61.

<u>If you try to go back on your own:</u>

You are running down the street following Trevor when you finally come to your senses. Sure, you followed your new friends into a dangerous situation. Sure, you panicked when you saw so much blood. But going back is the right thing.

"Trevor, wait. We need to go back!" Trevor slows down enough for you to catch up. "It's not too late to make a difference."

"No! No, I'm not going back. This is a disaster. I won't let anyone blame this mess on me!" he says.

You can't convince Trevor to go back. You stop running but Trevor continues toward home. You wander around trying to find the street where Eric lives, but you have no idea where it is.

<u>Continue on page 60.</u>

If you call 911, where will you tell the paramedics to go? Maybe someone else can convince Trevor to go back.

You call your mom. "Hi Mom, I need your help," you say in a shaky voice.

She can tell something isn't right. "What's wrong? she asks.

"Mom, I'm lost. I need to ping your phone with the address where I am, so you can come and pick me up."

Your mom gets the address and says, "Okay, I'll be right there."

When your mom picks you up, she can see that you are visibly shaken. Continue on page 62.

This is just terrible!"

Eric's mom continues, "There were injured people and blood everywhere. My son is having a severe stress reaction, but I understand he's the one who pulled the trigger. A horrible accident. My husband and the girl, Lisa were taken to the hospital. Since Trevor and his new friend were in the house, the police will be over to question them. I understand that Eric will be treated at the hospital for the trauma he went through and then taken into custody to be tried in juvenile court." [10]

Relief comes over you. You failed to do the right thing. You and Trevor weren't the least bit helpful when people were hurt. It's a good thing someone stepped up and got help when you were too scared to do anything.

You decide never to let anyone put you at risk again. After this, you know that if just one person stops to help, it can be the difference between life and death.

You also learn that everyone handles a dangerous situation differently. It's called fight or flight. You, Trevor and the others panicked and got out of there, which is okay, but at least one of you should have made sure to call for help first. * See picture on page 64. [6]

The End

You fill your mom in about the shooting and the emergency at Eric's house. Your mother is worried about you, because you're so upset.

"I'll be fine, mom. We need to go over to Trevor's house and tell his mom there's an emergency at Eric's house. Trevor knows where Eric lives, so he needs to call 911."

At Trevor's house, it takes both moms to convince him that he needs to report the accident and get help. Trevor is afraid he'll be blamed, but finally agrees.

You get into the neighbor's car and all four of you head back to Eric's house. This is such a disaster. Trevor has his phone on speaker and makes the call while his mother drives. You hear, "911 what's your emergency?"

Trevor says, "Kids were playing around with a gun and now some people have been shot."

Continue on page 63.

When you get to the house, the two who've been shot seem to be unconscious. There's so much bleeding.

"Are you at the house now?" the operator asks.

"Yes," Trevor says.

"Please stay on the line with me, help is on the way. Now will you tell me what you see?" she asks. "How many people are hurt?"

"Just Eric's dad and Lisa are hurt, I don't think Eric's hurt. He's walking around, but he's covered with blood."

"Okay, the two who are hurt may be critical," the operator says.

Trevor turns off the speaker but continues to listen to the 911 operator. "The operator wants us to find a piece of cloth to tie a tourniquet for both injured people," Trevor says.

Trevor's mom is running around in a panic. Your mom goes upstairs to find a bed sheet. You help your mother tear the sheet and make tourniquets to slow down the bleeding.

Continue on page 65.

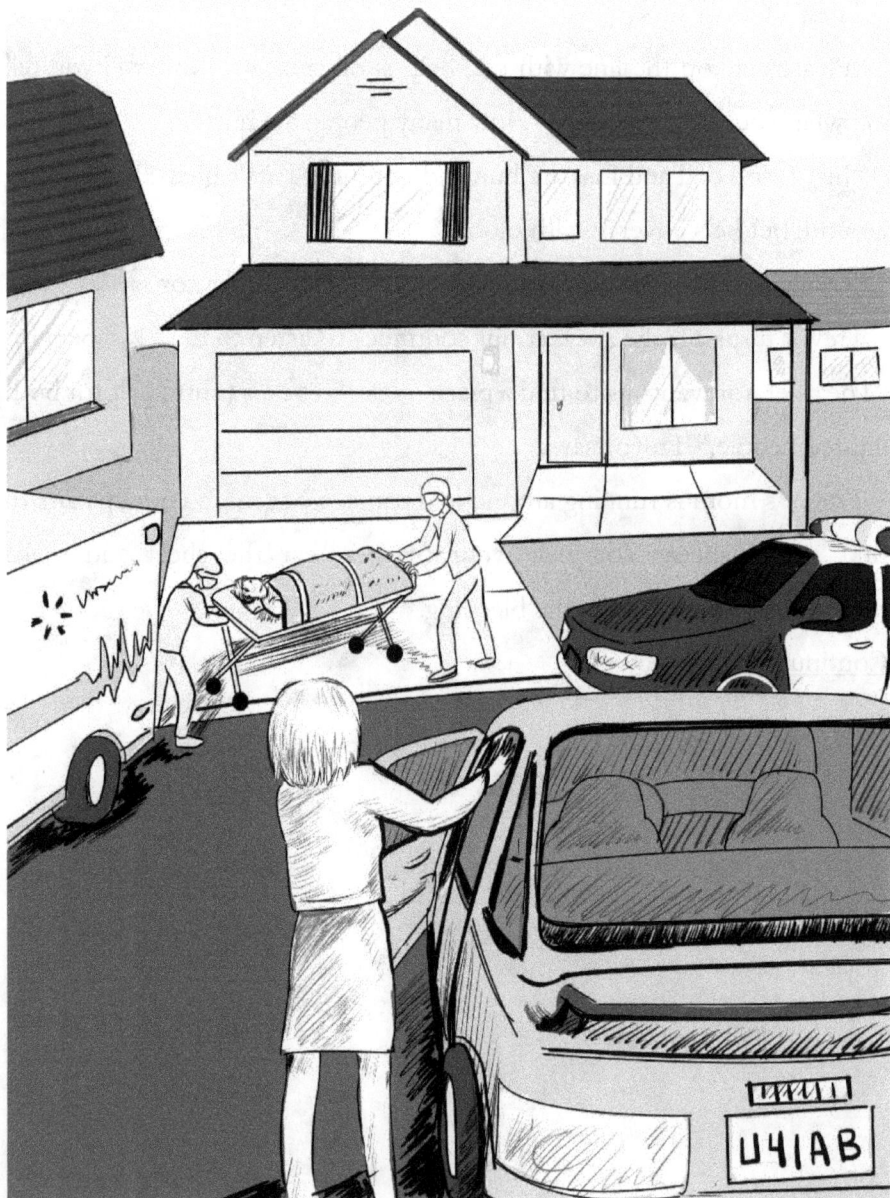

Six Kids, One Gun--

The paramedics arrive, but before they can enter the house, the police come in to secure the gun. An officer puts on gloves and lifts the weapon into an evidence bag. "All clear!" he says to the paramedics.

When the paramedics enter the home, one medic turns to Eric and says, "Your dad has a very weak heartbeat. He has lost too much blood."

You realize that because they were left for so long, Eric's dad could die. An officer tells the group, "Lisa is doing better, but if she was left much longer, she too would bleed out. A non-deadly wound can become deadly if left untreated," the officer says.

As soon as they are stabilized, the paramedics move the two wounded people to stretchers.

Eric's mom comes home and sees an ambulance, two fire trucks and two police cars in front of her house. She stops her car a few houses away and arrives in time to see the two injured people, including her husband, being taken out to the ambulance. "What, what happened?" she shrieks?" Your mother goes outside and explains, "There has been an accident with a gun. No one has been killed but your husband and Lisa need to be taken to the hospital. It would be best if you don't go inside the house right now until we clean things up." [34]

Continue on page 70.

"I, I'm new in town. I have no idea where I am. I know the guy who had the gun is Eric, but I don't know his last name."

The 911 operator tells you, "I have traced your location through your phone. Now I want you to find something tight and tie a tourniquet just above the area where the people were shot. This will slow down the bleeding."

The operator stays on the line with you. You find a tee shirt in Eric's room and cut it with a pair of kitchen scissors. Then you tie it just above each wound.

"Okay, I tied the tourniquets," you say.

"Thank you," she says, "Please stay on the line. "Help is on the way."

Eric asks you, "What happened?" He's conscious but not acting right. He seems to have no memory of the shooting.

You tell Eric, "The gun went off and it could have killed someone. I called 911 and help is on the way."

Eric looks around. He starts to realize what has happened and begins to panic. "I shot my dad and Lisa? Oh—I think I'm sick." He throws up on the already blood covered floor.

Continued on page 67

You're still on the phone with the .911 operator. She wants to talk to Eric. You hand your phone to him. You only hear Eric's side of the conversation and it's hard to know what the operator is asking him.

"Uh huh, uh huh. No, I'm not hurt. Yes, I think so. No, I didn't. No. I would never do that. Oh, my dad is right here but he can't talk right now.

"No, no. He's not. A girl. Lisa. Yes, she's hurt. No, she can't talk."

Eric hands the phone back to you. The operator tells you the police and ambulance have arrived. She says you can hang up now.

They come to the door and you open it. The first officer radios to someone saying, "We have an accidental shooting situation here. There are two down. I repeat, two down. We will need immediate medical assistance." The paramedics come in and check the two wounded people.

A paramedic says, "The man has been shot in the leg, and the girl in the shoulder.

Continue on page 68.

They're still alive, but the male, about thirty-five, five-foot ten is shot in the upper leg and has lost a lot of blood. Both seem stable and need to be taken to the nearest hospital."

Lisa rouses, not remembering what happened to her. The paramedics check her vital signs and her wound. The gunshot wound isn't critical. Lisa and Eric's dad are put on stretchers and wheeled out to the ambulance. *See picture on page 64

The paramedics also check Eric and take him to the hospital to treat him for traumatic stress.

You call your mom to let her know what happened and sit back down on the steps, stunned that a fun situation could turn deadly in just minutes.

Your mom is crying and scared. She doesn't know where to find you, but the cop talks to her on the phone. You hear him ask your mom for permission to get your statement. She must have said it was okay. He then tells her he'll take you home. You give your address.

You talk to the officer and tell him everything you know. "There were six kids in the house. No parents were home at the time Eric showed all of us the gun." [35]

Continue on page 69.

You continue giving your statement to the officer. "The weapon was in the nightstand where his mother kept it in case of an emergency. The kids were all excited about seeing and holding a gun. I knew it was loaded, but I was just as curious as the rest of the kids. The other kids ran off. Maybe they thought they were in trouble."

The police officer takes you home. Your mother runs to the car just as you are getting out. She hugs you. "I'm so glad you're safe!"

You see Trevor looking out the window at you and the officer. You wonder if you really want a friend like that. It seems like it would be better not to have a friend at all, then one who runs away when things get tough. You notice that the officer is heading over to Trevor's house to question him about the shooting.

Your parents sit you down. Your mother says, "Everyone handles a crisis in a different way. Trevor ran away in a panic because he was afraid and didn't know what to do."

Continue on page 73.

Trevor's mom drives Eric's mom to the hospital. On the way, they plan to pick up Lisa's mother.

You are asked to wait outside until the crime scene is cleared. Once the crime tape is removed, you help your mom and Trevor to clean up the blood from Eric's home.

When the cleanup is done, you call your dad, "Dad, we need you to come and pick us up at Eric's house. I will ping you the address. There has been an accident. Yes, mom and I are okay."

When your dad arrives, you and your mom fill him in on the accidental shooting. Your dad is shaking when he hears what has happened. You can tell he's trying to control his anger when he says, "this is just horrible! What were you thinking? You just moved here and now you are telling me that you and your new friends have been handling a loaded gun? It could have been you bleeding out on the living room floor! Then who would call 911? No one would even know your last name or where you live."

You and Trever mumble an apology. Trevor comes home with your family until his mom gets home.

You can hardly sleep that night. Your mom lets you stay home from school the next day. Eric is treated for a severe stress reaction. He has no wounds from the gun.

Eric's dad, though weak from the loss of blood, will survive his leg wound. Lisa is treated for a non-critical wound to her shoulder and released from the hospital the same night.

Continue on page 71.

Even though Eric's dad is shot, he is the registered gun owner so when he gets better, he could be charged for negligence in storing a weapon. He can also be charged with keeping a loaded gun in reach of a minor and the accidental shooting of the weapon by a minor. [27]

Eric is distraught. "I can't believe I not only shot my dad, but I also shot one of my close friends. Now my father could be taken to jail after he recovers from his wounded leg." As he is being taken away in handcuffs, he yells, "Lock me up! Lock me up! I did this! I'm guilty!"

Eric is taken to juvenile detention overnight. If he's charged with discharge of a weapon and causing injury, he could be held in detention, charged as an adult, or held in a diversion program for six months. [28] You and the other kids aren't arrested for the shooting.

You know all this could have been prevented if you would have just told someone about the gun. [7], [4], [12]

The End

Eric stands up. The counselor continues, "I want to speak with your parents in the morning, along with the parents of the boys who pick on you. I'll make some phone calls right away. Eric, you *will* get help here, I promise. The boys will possibly face termination. Your parent's may also decide to take the case to court. You're not alone, and I certainly don't want you to become desperate enough to hurt someone."

You've remained outside the door and heard the whole conversation.

Eric sees you when he leaves the office and gives you a slight smile. "Did you tell?" He asks you.

Continue on page 78.

Your dad says, "You handled a terrible situation better and more calmly than most kids would. I really think they should have drills at school, teaching kids what to do in case of an emergency."

The next day at school, you try to avoid Trevor and his questions. You notice that Eric and Sara aren't at school. After school lets out, you ask your mom to take you to the hospital, so you can see if Eric's dad is okay. When you walk into the hospital room, Eric's dad is conscious, and he's visiting with his wife and son.

Eric's dad says, "There's our hero! You're the one who saved our lives! When everyone else ran away, you stayed right there and called 911! The doctors tell me that timing is critical with a gunshot wound. [*3] People can even die from a leg or a shoulder wound. The main thing is to get help before someone can bleed out. Here I am, alive and well because help arrived quickly. It still required several hours of surgery, to put me back together."

You don't really consider yourself to be a hero. You only know that you stayed when the others ran off. You also know that if you had told someone about the gun sooner, none of this would have happened.

Continue on page 75.

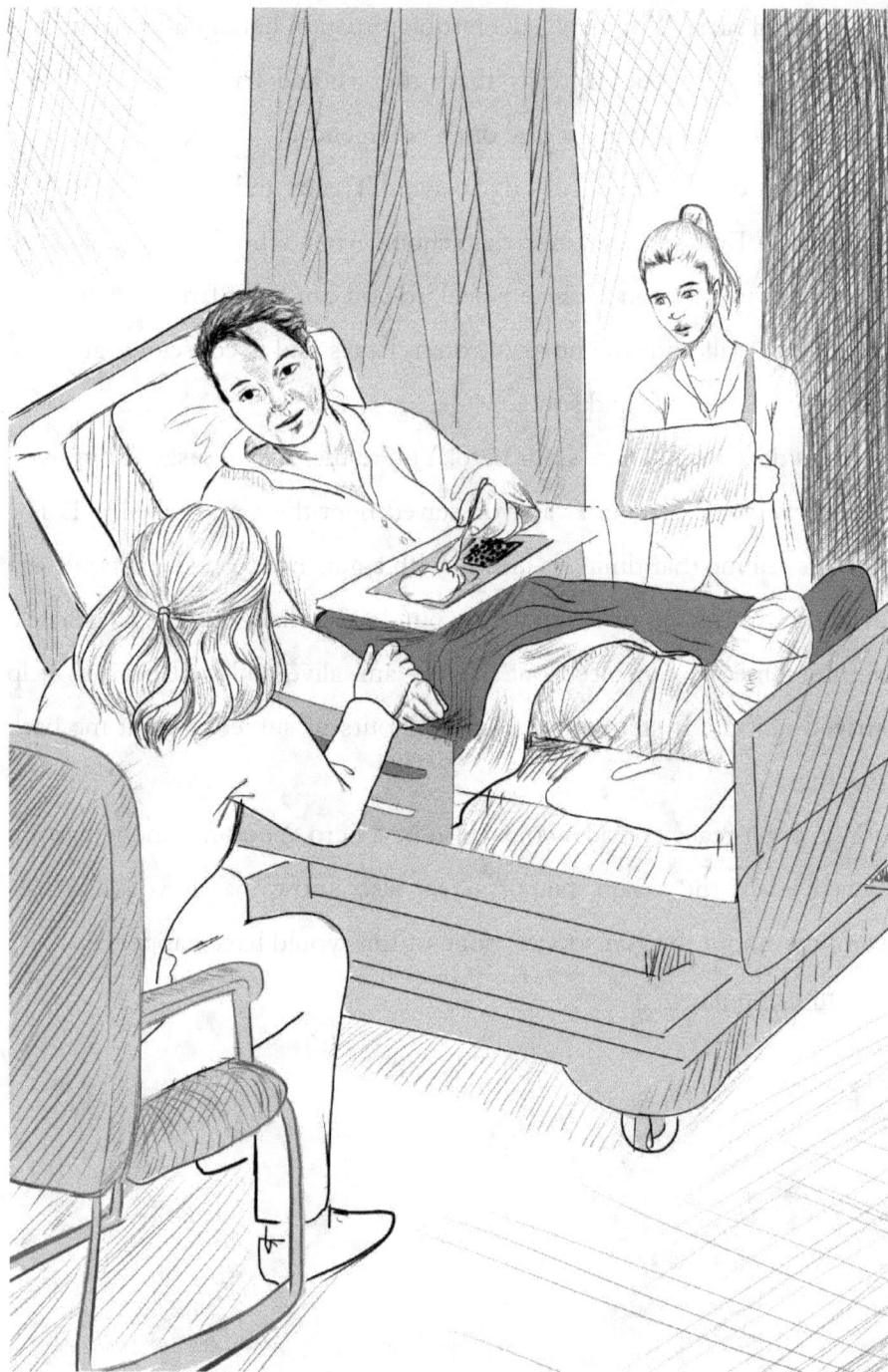

Lisa walks into the hospital room, wearing a sling.

"There she is," Eric's dad says. "How're you doing?"

"My wound wasn't serious. The bullet went right through my arm and ended up in the wall by the steps. I was treated for my injury at the hospital and released the same day."

"That's great!" you say.

Eric is charged with illegal possession of a firearm, discharge of a weapon and causing injury. The juvenile court system is designed to give rehab to juveniles committing crimes, while the adult justice system gives penalties. In some cases, minors can be charged as adults. Eric could get probation for his crimes, go to a diversion program for six months or spend time in a detention center. [*4]

Continue on page 76.

In some states the law says the homeowner is responsible in the case of an accidental shooting with a firearm that has not been properly stored in a place that is safely away from minors. In this case, the gun was registered to Eric's dad. Once he recovers, Eric's dad, even though he was shot, could be charged with a crime and even serve jail time. [*5]

You know that Eric's dad has been shot and that it was an accident. You also know that the others didn't run to get help, even though they knew two people were shot. You wonder what kind of friends would do that? Trevor, your neighbor and new friend panicked and didn't even stay to see if everyone was okay.

Your dad explains to you that "everyone reacts differently when faced with an emergency. The way the others reacted was a normal reaction to fear. We are so proud of you for staying calm and getting help in this terrible situation."

The End

Eric admits, "I've never shot a gun before, but my dad bought the targets, so he could show me how to shoot."

Eric goes first. He hits a target in the lower body where it gives him seven points. For his next shot, he hits the same target high on the silhouette body and earns another seven points.

Everyone says: "Aww!" You give him a high five.

Trevor's turn is next. He aims at the target and hits a bottle, which fragments. Everyone says "Oh-h-h!"

On his next shot he once again aims at the target but hits a rose bush—scattering red petals all around. He quits because he can't seem to hit the target. Trevor hands the gun over to you.

What should you do? It's time to choose a path:

If you refuse to shoot the gun—continue on page 82.

If you take your turn and shoot the gun—continue on page 85.

You nod. He gives you a weak, "thank you." And whispers in your ear. "I have a gun."

A chill runs down your spine.

Eric doesn't even go to his locker before going home.

Just for bringing a gun to school, even if Eric decided not to show the gun, or shoot it, he could be charged as an adult with a weapons charge. He could get a substantial prison sentence. [24] His life and all his future plans would come to a sudden halt and he'd be a prisoner, serving alongside other much older criminals.

You would never see him in school again.

The End

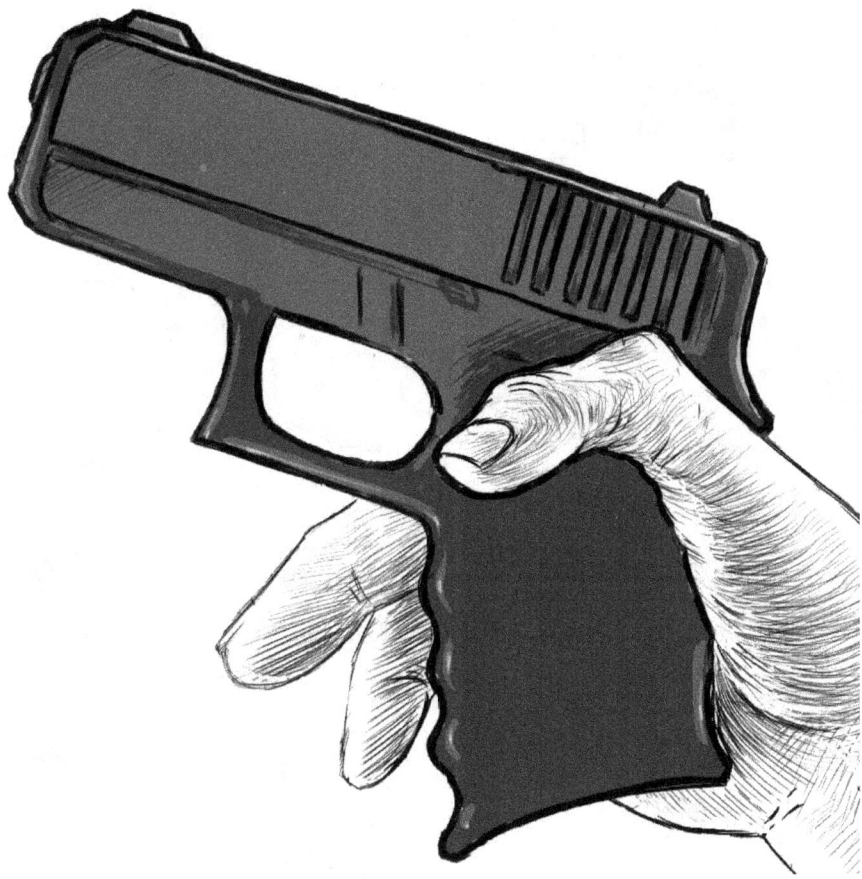

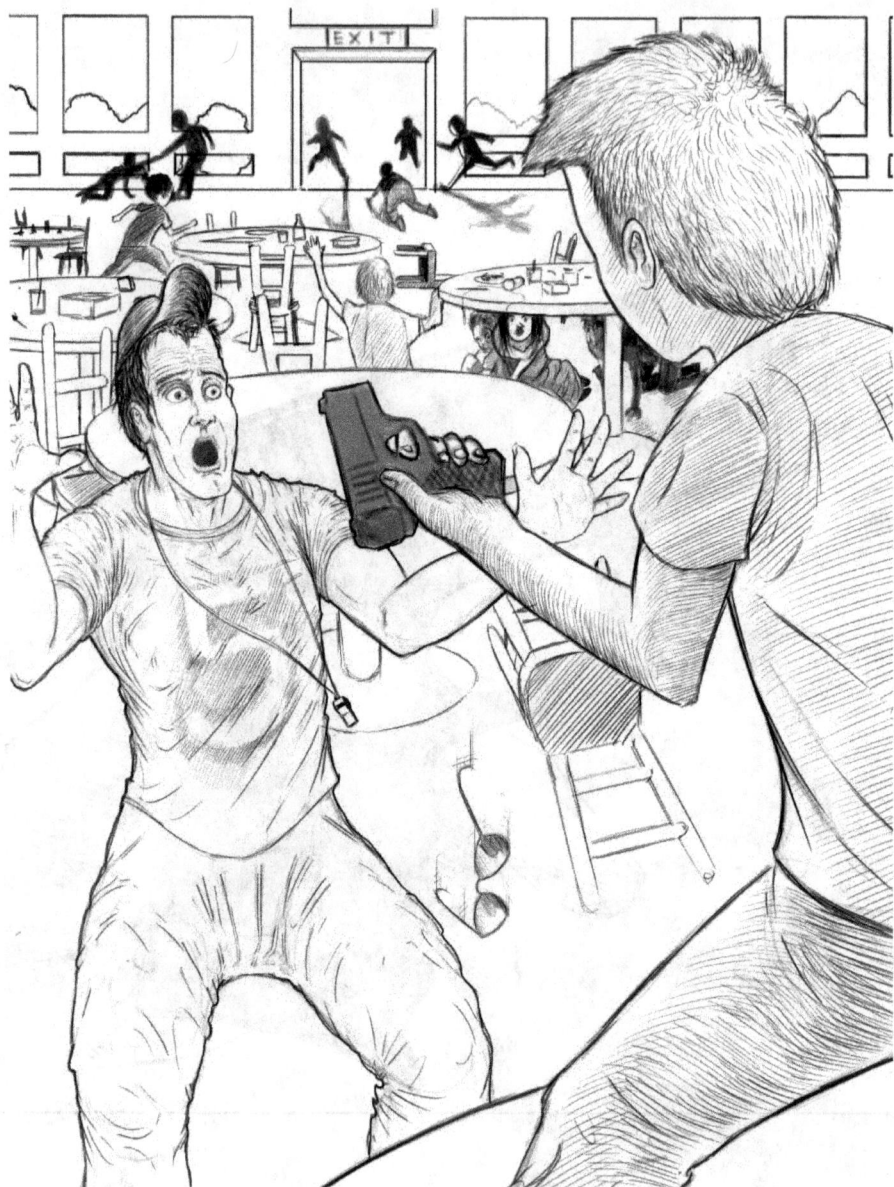

If Eric takes the gun to school

While in the office, you have second thoughts about going home on your second day. You leave the office and go to your next class.

When you meet your new group of friends for lunch, Eric seems agitated and fidgety. The group of guys who bully him enter the room. Eric doesn't even wait for them to get close to his table. He stands up on the bench in the cafeteria and pulls out the gun. "Who do you think is in charge here?" he asks. "Well it certainly isn't you!" he shouts to the guys on the football team. He's sweaty and loud. You wonder if he's been drinking.

Eric continues to bring drama to the situation. He shoots a warning round into the ceiling, and everyone ducks. Girls are screaming, the football jocks try to escape the room.

Eric shouts, "Don't think you can just leave. You've made my life miserable. Don't you think that gives me the right to make your life just as unhappy?"

An announcement comes over the intercom, "Students and teachers, we have a lockdown situation. Do not enter the cafeteria at this time. Please enter the nearest classroom. No one enters or leaves this school. This is a lockdown situation"

Continue on page 84.

If you refuse to shoot the gun

You watch Eric and Trevor shoot the gun. You're beginning to see that shooting a gun in an open backyard is very harmful.

You speak up, "I really don't think it's a good idea to shoot a gun out in the open. Someone could get hurt." You begin to back away from the gun. No one seems to agree with you. They're still waiting for a turn to pull the trigger.

Tyler says, "If you don't want to shoot, then it's my turn."

You walk away, into the front yard and call your mom. When she answers you say, "Mom, I should have told you sooner, but the kids I'm hanging out with are all at Eric's house, shooting a gun in the backyard."

Your mother is alarmed. You ping her phone, so she knows your location and she calls 911. Your mom puts her phone on Bluetooth and stays on the line with the operator, while driving to Eric's house. An officer and your mom arrive at about the same time. You show them to the backyard. The kids you were hanging out with are laughing and joking around.

Continue on page 91.

My dog's been shot!" the owner, who lives at a nearby house is hollering. You hear a lot of commotion, but you don't come out of hiding.

Eric tells everyone to come out of hiding, as the dog owner runs down the street, carrying her dog! "Call animal control," says the owner. "My dog's been shot."

From your hiding place in the garage, you can hear kids running and hear the shouts of alarm about the dog that's been shot. Eric gets all the other kids to go into the house. You're still hiding in the garage and you're not coming out. One by one, you see cars arrive and the parents of the kids involved enter the house where Eric lives.

You go to the garage window and watch what's going on outside.

The police arrive and begin to question the neighborhood kids. Someone says, "I think the shots came from that house," and the boy points to Eric's house.

Continue on page 96.

The football coach comes in and talks Eric into giving up the gun. "I know the guys are really tough on you, Eric. If you shoot someone, you'll never have a better life. Please, son, give up the gun before someone gets hurt."

Eric, hands over the gun. The school security come in, along with the police, who put handcuffs on Eric. One officer reads Eric his Miranda Rights. "Eric Brown, you have the right to remain silent. Anything you say can and will be used against you in a court of law. You have the right to an attorney. If you cannot afford an attorney, one will be provided for you. [33]

The girls are crying, and your group of kids tell Eric they will testify against the bullies.

You know for sure that Eric won't return to school this year.

In some states minors have been tried as adults for bringing a weapon to school and discharging a weapon on school property. If he's tried as a minor, Eric could remain in custody and serve in a juvenile detention center up to the age of twenty-one. [26]

If only you and your new friends had listened to the gut feeling that Eric would bring the gun to school, someone could have prevented this serious situation.

The End

If you take your turn and shoot the gun

It's your turn to shoot the gun. You aim at the target and hit the edge of a different target. You try again but the next bullet doesn't seem to hit anything. Off in a distance, you hear a crash. You all look around and find that the bullet has hit a window in the house behind Eric's house. The window is shattered.

There's a scream from the house where the bullet hit. A mother runs through a side door with her child wrapped in a blanket. "Who shot at my daughter, asleep in her bed?" she hollers, "Call the police! Someone call 911! A bullet went through the window and barley missed my child!"

Eric grabs the gun and runs into his house, saying, "I need to put the gun away, quick so it can't be traced back to me." All your friends follow him into the house.

Continue on page 87.

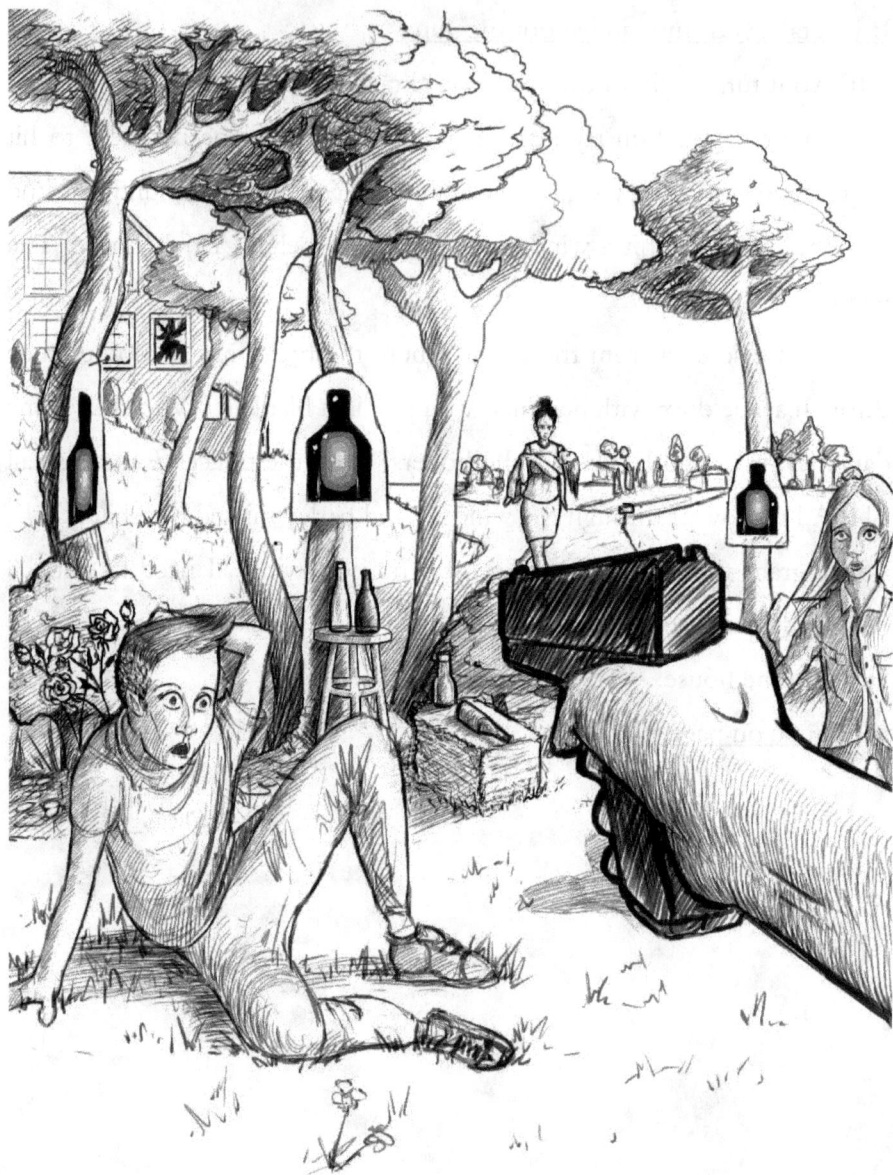

You're stunned! You try to run but you can't even walk. You're standing there in the same spot you stood when a bullet from the gun *you shot* hit a window. Thoughts are racing through your mind. I didn't aim at a child. How did that happen? It isn't my gun. It isn't even my backyard.

What should you do? It's time to choose a path:

If you turn yourself in for the shooting—continue on page 90.

If you run into Eric's house to hide—continue on page 88.

If you run into Eric's house to hide:

You had a turn to shoot the gun, and you really messed up. You follow Eric, Trevor, Tyler, Sara and Lisa into the house. When you get inside, Eric goes upstairs, and you follow. You want to make sure, once and for all that Eric puts the gun back into the drawer. Now what? A lady is running down the street with a scared child. You nearly shot the child with a stray bullet and all you can do is run into the house like a chicken.

Trevor says, "Eric, it's just a matter of time until someone finds out that our new friend here," he motions toward you, "shot the gun through the window. You'd better call your dad, dude. He'll know what to do."

"No, I can't," Eric says. "We weren't supposed to be playing with the gun."

"Okay," Trevor says, "I'll call my dad then."

"No! No, you can't," Eric says, grabbing Trevor by the arm. Eric seems so frightened.

You're visibly shaking. This is the first time you've ever shot a gun, and you nearly kill a kid. You take out your cell phone and text your mom. She'll know what to do.

Continue on page 89.

Mom, I went with Trevor to a guy named Eric's house. Eric had a gun. We were doing target practice in the backyard. A bullet I shot went through a window and it nearly hit a little girl. I don't know what to do. The police are on their way here and we're all hiding inside the house. Eric won't call his dad. Mom, I think I'm in trouble. Help!

There's no more joking around at Eric's house now. The police arrive, and you think they've already traced the bullet to Eric's backyard. They knock at the door, but Eric pulls you back from the window.

"I want to go to the door and confess," you say.

"No," Eric says. "I think you'll go to jail for attempted murder!" [15]

This really upsets you. Everyone in the house is silent. You hear one of the officer's say he's going door to door until he finds out the name and location of the homeowner.

The ambulance arrives with sirens blaring and takes the woman and her child to the hospital. Now you aren't sure if the child was hurt, but earlier you heard the mother say the bullet didn't hit her child.

Continue on page 98.

You realize that if you run into Eric's house, the police will find you anyway. If you hurry up and take down all the evidence of target practice, someone will see you running around in the backyard.

Other thoughts race through your head. A child has nearly been shot, and I'm responsible. If I run home, the police will find me. It's my fault! If only I had reported the gun yesterday, today I wouldn't have found myself in this situation. Why did I let fear of losing my new friendships take over and cloud my mind? I could've talked to Trevor, to Eric, or my parents. Why, oh why didn't I?

You start to worry about being put on trial for attempted murder. I could be tried as an adult. I'm still a kid and not ready to give up my whole future. *11

Then your thoughts go back to the little kid. Her mother is running down the street in a panic, trying to get someone to call 911 and get help for a frightened child. A child who could have been shot. Killed! A child who might not have grown up, because you shot a gun. A child who won't be the same. She should've always felt safe in her own home. She shouldn't have to be afraid to sleep in her own bed. You did this, and you know it.
Continue on page 92.

Two more kids have shot at the target while you were waiting for your mom. Eric has the gun in his hand again. He's pretending to shoot at each target and bottle. Just as you're entering the backyard with the officer, the gun goes off with a loud bang. Eric shoots at a bottle and it shatters into tiny pieces.

"Hold it right there," the police officer says. "Son, put down the firearm, and slowly back away."

"That's it. Slowly now."

"Who owns this gun, son?" he asks Eric.

"Uh, my parents," Eric says.

"Did you know that it's illegal for a minor to have possession of a firearm? And to be shooting a firearm in a populated area?"

"Uh, no."

"It's also illegal for a minor to shoot a firearm without supervision."

"Uh-oh," Eric says.

"I need to talk to your parents, son."

Eric calls his parents and they arrive shortly.

Continue on page 94.

You've just become the monster that comes to scare little kids.

There's a voice inside your head, saying "Do the right thing." Now you're the only one who can handle this. All the other kids have run away. They're hiding inside the house. You know the cops can trace the path of the bullet to Eric's house. Eric brought out the gun. His parents own the gun, but you, you shot at a kid, asleep in her bed.

Someone must've called 911 because the police and an ambulance arrive quickly. The child and her mom are checked over and taken in the ambulance.

Now you start to panic. Maybe the child *was* shot. You aren't sure, but she went into the ambulance with her mother.

You hurry to the back of Eric's yard, into the yard where the bullet hit. You walk down the driveway, sweating and shaking. You go up to the police officer and tell him in a shaky voice. "I did it."

Continue on page 93.

You're talking so quietly that the officer can't understand what you said. "I, I did this. I shot the gun."

The officer bends down slightly and repeats your words back to you as a question. "You're saying that you had a gun and you shot through the window and nearly harmed a child?"

You're visibly shaking, and your mouth has gone dry. "Yes, I shot the gun. I have never shot a gun before and it was an accident."

The officer is completely still for a moment, as if trying to process what you just told him. "You're saying that you shot a gun, and have never shot a gun before?"

"Yes."

"We need to call one of your parents," he says.

You call your mother and the officer tells her the address for Eric's house.

When your mother arrives, the officer begins to question you. "Where did you get the gun?" he asks you.

"My friend had a gun." [*29]

Continue on page 95.

When Eric's dad arrives, the officer questions him about the gun. He also writes out a citation for him to appear before a judge. He's told that it's not only illegal for a minor to have possession of a firearm, it's also illegal to shoot a gun in a populated area.

All the kid's parents are called, and the officer waits until they arrive before questioning the kids.

An officer reads the Miranda Rights and Eric and the others who shot the gun, are handcuffed and taken to juvenile detention. [41] In the juvenile system, they could get detention, probation, put into a diversion program or be given community service. [14]

It's possible you won't be seeing your new friends for quite a while. You're glad you didn't shoot the gun. You did the right thing, trying to stop this before anyone got hurt. [36, 37]

The End

"Where is your friend now and where's the gun?"

Before you can answer, a second officer, who was checking the crime scene, comes back and says, "I found the path of the bullet. Come over here. There are several targets set up and several spent bullets."

"You come with me," says the first officer who was questioning you. You and your mom follow to the fence of Eric's yard.

After seeing evidence of the shooting, the officer you spoke to says, "It's time we spoke with the homeowner." He walks around to Eric's front door and knocks. You continue to follow. Kids' peek out through the curtains, but no one answers the door.

"Dispatch," the officer says into his radio. "Will you find the homeowner for the following address? We need a phone number where he can be reached." He then recites Eric's address. Eric's dad is located and arrives home shortly.

The officer tells Eric's dad what took place at his home while he was away. His dad is shown the targets and bottles set up in his backyard.

"Sir, do you own a gun?"

Continue on page 100.

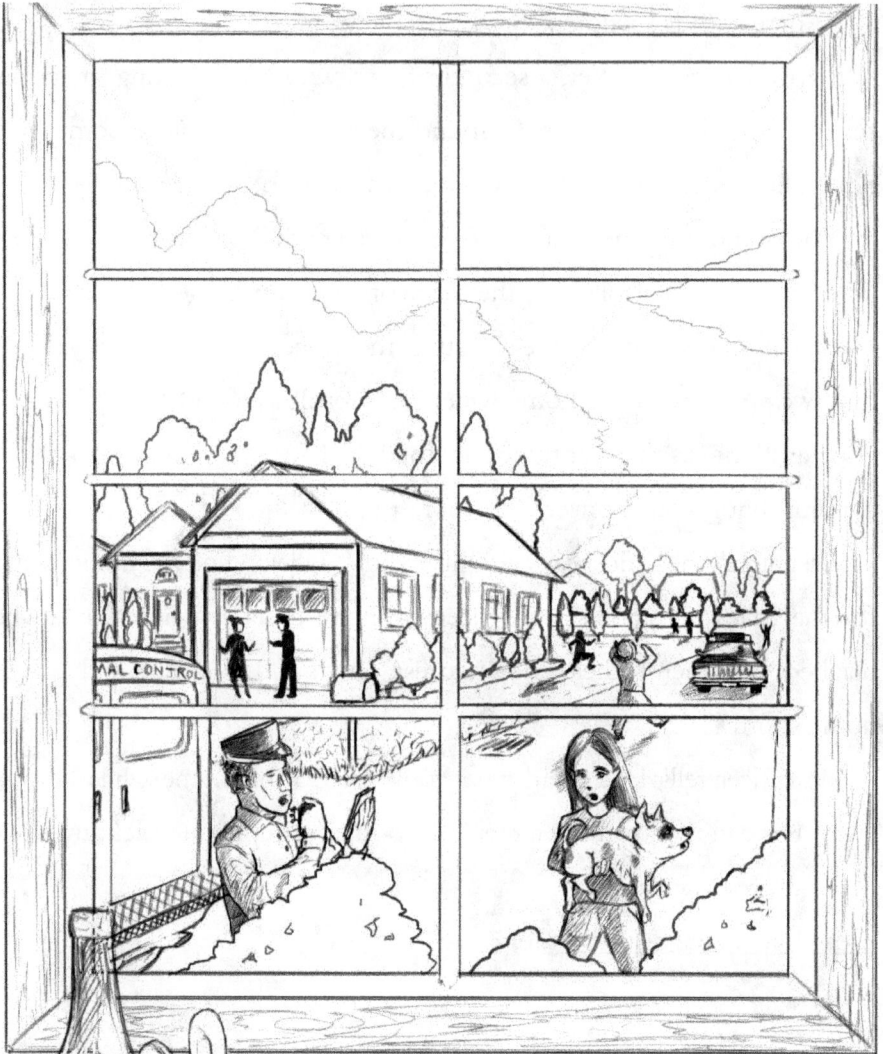

An officer knocks on Eric's door. You can see the officer talking to Lisa in the doorway to the house. She comes outside and says, "Our friend is shot! I'm sure someone must have shot our friend!" She explains to the officer what happened and that you're now missing and must've been shot. There's a moment of panic from your group as they think you've been shot. Trevor tries to describe you for the officer. The police scour the area. Trevor must've called his parents because both his and your parents arrive and assist the police in looking for you. You're so shaken up that you really don't want to be found.

When you're found in the garage, your parents are so relived! They hug you and your mom kisses you in front of all your friends. Mom asks if they can take you home. A police officer tells her he needs to get your statement.

"Hey everyone, I'm okay. I didn't get shot. I just got scared when Eric was shooting the gun," you say.

Continue on page 108.

The police must've located Eric's dad because a short time later, Eric's dad and your mom arrive.

Eric's dad opens the door to the house and says, "The police already know someone from the house shot the bullet that went through a window. Eric, you and your friends need to come out here, right now, and talk to the police."

One by one the kids go outside, and you follow. Eric's dad then runs into the house followed by a police officer, he goes upstairs and returns outside with the officer carrying the firearm.

Your mom is there. Each of the other kids are told to call their parents.

As each parent arrives, the officers question their teen.

"The gun has been shot recently. If we test the bullet that went through the window, against the ones in your backyard, I can guarantee that they came from this gun," an officer says.

Continue on page 99.

Another officer says, "The targets and the bottles set up in the yard are a dead giveaway. I don't think we need to test anything here."

"Okay, young people, who shot this gun?"

No one moves for a moment, then Sara nudges you from behind.

"Okay, then, we'll test all of you for gunpowder," the first officer says.

Because of your text, your mother knows you're the one who shot through the window. She puts her arm around you and brings you forward so you can talk to the officer. "I did it. It was my turn to shoot the gun. I've never shot a gun before. The first bullet hit the target on the tree, but the second bullet didn't seem to hit anything. Then we all heard the window back there break and we were pretty sure the bullet hit the window. When the lady came out of the house saying I almost hit a child, we all panicked and ran into the house,"

"We can see that this was an accident, but there are several illegal infractions here. One, the homeowner failed to lock up a firearm, two, the gun was loaded and in easy access to a minor.

Continue on page 102.

"Yes, actually I own several, but they're locked up in my gun safe."

"Is it possible that you have a gun that isn't locked up? Or maybe someone in your household knows the combination?"

"No, well we do keep a gun in the nightstand, in case of emergency. I don't think anyone has ever shot that gun. Just a moment, I'll go check to see if the gun is still there." The second officer follows Eric's dad as he runs upstairs to get the gun.

They walk down the stairs and come back outside. The second officer, who followed him, is now carrying the gun.

The officer examines the gun and then says. "As I suspected, this gun has been fired recently."

Eric's dad shakes his head. "I had no idea."

You're still standing next to the cops. They haven't put you in handcuffs, so maybe that's a good sign.

The second officer, holding the gun says, "I can almost bet that if we pick up the bullets in the backyard and also the one that went through the window of the house behind you, it will match this gun."

Continue on page 101.

The first officer, who was questioning you before asks, "Is this the gun you were shooting in the backyard?"

You say, "Yes."

While the second officer searches around the outside of the house for evidence and the first is writing in a notepad, Eric's dad looks at you suspiciously. "Now, who are you?"

"I-I just met Eric yesterday. I'm new in town."

"You weren't here alone, shooting my gun in the backyard. Where's Eric?"

You say, "He was here with some other kids, but they all ran into the house. I think they got scared and they must be hiding."

Eric's dad shakes his head in disbelief. "They just left you to take all the blame?"

"Well, I'm the one who shot through the window," you say.

The first police officer than asks you, "How many other kids were shooting the gun?"

"Well, there were six kids, including me. Only two other kids shot the gun, before I shot through the window."

Continue on page 103.

The officer continues, "three, the gun was used in a populated area and without supervision. Four, if the bullet had hit and killed the child, it could have been involuntary manslaughter. As it is, since you missed the child you could be charged with reckless endangerment. [16]

You suck in a breath.

"Today young people, the three kids who shot the gun will be arrested and taken into custody of the Juvenile Justice System. You have the right to remain silent. Anything you say can and will be used against you in a court of law. You have the right to an attorney. If you cannot afford an attorney, one will be provided for you. Now, each of you will spend the night in detention and tomorrow you'll be seen by a judge," the officer says. Each of you are handcuffed and put into a police car.

The officer turns to the homeowner. "You could be charged with illegal discharge of a firearm and improper storage of a firearm and the discharge of a firearm by a minor." [17, 30]

Continue on page 105.

The second officer has returned and he's listening. "I think it's time to get those kids out here, don't you?" The other officer agrees.

"Open up, police, I need to ask you some questions."

Eric finally opens the door and walks out, followed by Trevor. "It's only the two of us here. We're the ones who shot the gun. The rest of the kids went home."

Trevor is told to call a parent as well. After his mother arrives the second officer takes Eric and Trevor and their parents aside to question them. You overhear part of the conversation. Eric says, "Yes, I took out the gun, but I didn't shoot at a little kid!"

Returning to his questions the first officer askes Eric's dad, "Sir, is this gun registered to you?"

"Yes."

"We'll need to bag the gun as evidence." He pulls an evidence bag out of the patrol car, marks it with a case number and the date and puts the gun inside.

Continue on 104.

An officer tells Eric's dad, "Well sir, I need you to come down to the station with me for questioning. At the very least, your gun was used by a minor in an unsecured residential area. The gun is registered to you and it was a loaded gun, improperly stored so a minor had easy access to the weapon. [12] You are not being arrested at this time."

You're very anxious to hear how the child is doing. While the first officer helps Eric's dad into the car, the second officer, after questioning Eric and Trevor, comes to talk to you. "The child has only suffered a few cuts from the broken glass. She's doing just fine."

Continue on page 106.

Even though you're being charged with a crime through the Juvenile Justice System, you won't be charged as an adult. You're likely to get probation, detention up to six months or community service for shooting a gun. [18]

You'll never forget that you shot a bullet that nearly hit a sleeping child. You also know that this could have been prevented if only you had spoken up—telling someone about the gun. [40]

See picture on page 107.

The End

You're so relieved that she's doing okay.

An officer says to all of you, "You are under arrest for handling and shooting a weapon. You have the right remain silent. Anything you say can and will be used against you in a court of law. You have the right to an attorney. If you cannot afford an attorney, one will be provided for you." [31]

You, Eric and Trevor are placed in handcuffs and escorted to the other police car. You're taken to juvenile detention to wait for a trial. If charged with illegal possession of a firearm, shooting in a residential area, and reckless endangerment, you could serve time in a detention center, be put into a diversion program for up to six months, be put on probation or be sentenced with community service. [13]

Why didn't you have the courage to speak up sooner? If the kid you nearly shot, someday forgets what happened or is too young to remember, you won't forget. You will always think about the day you accidentally shot at a little kid.

The End.

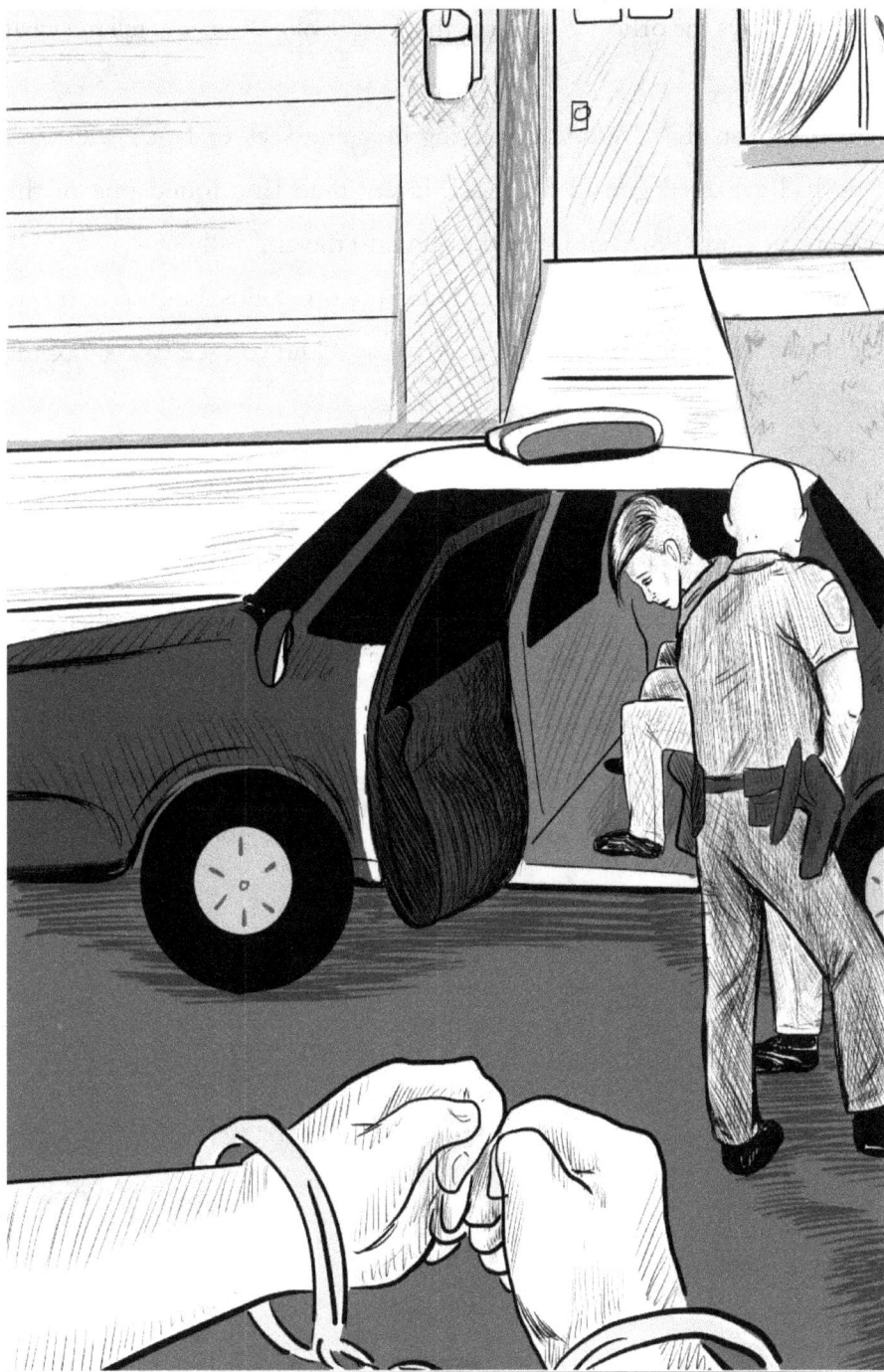

"Okay," says the officer. "I can see that you're okay. Can you tell me what happened?"

You explain that, "We were playing hide and seek in Eric's backyard. Eric had a loaded gun in his hand. Every time Eric found one of the players, he said, 'Pow,' and shot the gun into the air."

Another officer had already questioned the other kids, but both officers seem very interested in what you have to say. "Did you see Eric shoot the gun?"

"No," you say. "But I did see him bring the gun out of the house and every time he found someone, I heard his voice saying, 'pow.'" You continue: "When he made the last shot, I heard a dog yelp. After that, I looked out the window from the garage and saw a girl carrying her dog, saying the dog is shot."

"And then what happened?" the officer asks.

"I heard Eric running around finding the other kids. I think someone called Animal Protection and the police. Then Eric got all the kids back into the house."

"Why didn't you come out from hiding then?"

Continue on page 109.

"I was afraid. I knew the dog was shot. What if one of us *had* been shot? I was also afraid that Eric would go to jail."

"Thank you. You are free to go home with your parents," the officer says to you. "I'll be in touch if I have more questions."

"Eric Brown, you are going to be held in detention overnight and appear in juvenile court tomorrow," the officer says. He puts handcuffs on Eric and reads him the Miranda Rights. [30]

In the juvenile system, he could be charged with a weapons charge and for harming an animal. He could get detention, community service or be sentenced to a diversion or wilderness program for six months. In some cases, a juvenile can be charged as an adult and serve time in prison. [19]

Eric's dad could also be charged with improper storage of a firearm, and the use of a weapon by a minor without supervision. [20]

The gun is registered to Eric's dad. He's taken in for questioning. If found guilty for improper storing of a firearm, in some states parents are prosecuted for the crimes committed by minors who access their weapon. [21]

Continue on page 110

You and the other kids aren't being arrested. You realize that this was a close call. Someone could've really been shot. In this case, a dog was shot. No one should be shooting a gun in an unprotected area. You feel lucky that you weren't shot and know you should never play around with a gun.

You also find out that the dog has been injured and will require surgery. The homeowner—Eric's dad, will probably have to pay for the surgery as well as fines for the harm of the pet.[19, 38]

The End

Statistics from Gifford's Law Center to Prevent Gun Violence

Statistics on Gun Deaths & Injuries

- 31,076 Americans died in homicides, suicides and unintentional shootings in 2010. This equals more than 85 deaths per day and more than three deaths an hour.

- In homes where guns are kept unlocked and loaded, the risk of suicide increases.

Unintentional Deaths and Injuries

- Unintentional firearm injuries caused the deaths of 606 people in the year 2010.

- In a five-year period from 2005-2010, almost 3,800 people in the U.S. died from unintentional shootings.

- During that same period, over 1,300 victims of unintentional shootings were under 25 years of age.

- A federal study of unintentional shootings found that 8% of these shooting deaths resulted from shots fired by children under the age of six.

- The U.S. General Accounting Office estimates that 31% of unintentional firearm caused deaths might be prevented by the addition of a child-proof safety lock and a loading indicator

Statistics on Youth Gun Violence & Gun Access

- Each day in the US, 18 children and young adults (24 and under) die from firearm injuries.

- More than one third of all deaths and non-fatal firearm injuries are children and young adults (24 years of age and under).

111

- Around 4.6 million minors in the US live in homes with at least one loaded, unlocked firearm.

- More than 75% of guns used in suicide attempts and unintentional injuries of 0-19-year-olds were stored in the residence of the victim, a relative, or a friend.

- More than half of U.S. homes with children and firearms have one or more firearms without trigger locks in an unlocked place, according to a 2000 study.

- In another study, parents reported that their children age nine and under did not know the location of their firearm, while their children reported that they not only knew the location of the gun, but many of the children admitted to handling the weapon when their parents weren't home.

- 89% of accidental shooting deaths among children occur in the home and most of these deaths occur when children are playing with an unsecured loaded gun in their parents' absence.

- The practices of keeping firearms locked, unloaded, and storing ammunition in a locked location separate from firearms may assist in reducing youth suicide and unintentional injury in homes with children and teenagers where guns are stored.

- Even children as young as three years old, are strong enough to fire a handgun.

Each Life

That is Ended

Through

Gun Violence,

Suicide or

Accidental Death

Leaves Behind

A Million

Broken

Hearts

References

If you think you might be in trouble with the law, your parents should get you a lawyer—there are lawyers who specialize in juvenile cases. If you can't afford a lawyer, one will be assigned to you in court.

If you feel suicidal or if you know someone who is suicidal—call or have them call the **United States National Suicide and Crisis Hotline— Open 24 hours a day: Talk 1-800-273-8255 or Suicide 1-800-784-2433**

To report an incident with a gun, call 911. If you suspect someone has a gun at school or you overhear a conversation or see a post on the internet—talk to someone. It's not safe to talk to the person with the gun, so report it to a parent, teacher, school security or the police. Hoping for the best is not a plan!

Fun, not guns!

There's plenty to do to keep kids busy these days. I suggest fun, not guns! To find an extensive list of things for kids to do, go to my website at this link: https://www.jillvanderwood.com/dmyu/bored.html

If you are being bullied, there are many ways to handle the situation: Here are some resources:

Are you a victim of crime? National Center for Victims of Crime: http://www.ncvc.org or office of Victims of Crime: http://www.ovc.org

Are you gay or think you might be gay? Gay Lesbian and Straight Education Network: http://www.glsen.org

Ask the Judge: Answers for teens about the law: http://www.askthejudge.info/

Breaking Down Barriers: The Chris Hendrick Band perform and speaks to youth about bullying: http://www.chrishendricksmusic.com/

Bullies to Buddies, the simple solution to bullying:

http://www.bullies2buddies.com/

Byparents-forParents.com

Dealing with bullying: Kid Health.org,
http://www.kidshealth.org/teen/your_mind/problems/bullies.html

Erase the Problem of Bullying: (book or Kindle book) by Jill Ammon
Vanderwood
https://www.amazon.com/Erase-Problem-Bullying-Ammon-Vanderwood/

Human Rights Campaign: http://www.hrc.org

Kid Power: http://www.kidpower.org/bullying/

Stomp out Bullying: http://www.stompotbullyin.org

Stop Bullying.gov: What is bullying, cyberbullying? Who's at risk? Prevent
bullying: http://www.stopbullying.gov/

Stop Bullying Now organization:
http://www.stopbullyingnowfoundation.org/main

Violence Prevention Works, the world's foremost bullying prevention
program: http://www.violencepreventionworks.org/public.page

Sources for Off Target

*1 Laws for Criminal Liability when a Child Gains Access as a Result of Negligent Storage of a Firearm:

Fourteen states and the District of Columbia have laws that impose criminal liability on persons who negligently store firearms, where minors could or do gain access to the firearm. http://lawcenter.giffords.org/gun-laws/policy-areas/child-consumer-safety/child-access-prevention/

*2 Criminal Weapons Possessions Laws apply to both adults and juveniles. Most of the time, minors are sent through the juvenile court system, where the aim is to counsel and rehabilitate, rather than punish the offender. Juvenile Weapons Possession By Mark Theoharis https://www.criminaldefenselawyer.com/resources/juvenile-weapons-possession.htm

*3 Will you die after being shot in the leg/arm?

You can die from being shot in the arm or leg, but it largely depends on how long it takes for you to get medical attention. The most likely causes of death from a gunshot wound to an extremity are bleeding out and infection. Quora—Tara Nitka

*4 Warning, Community service, or Diversion. These programs require the juvenile to spend 6 months or so, participating programs for community service, or other programs designed to rehabilitate the child. Probation. Probation usually lasts at least 6 months and the juvenile is required to obey court orders to stay out of trouble, stay in school or to keep a job. Juvenile Weapons Possession By Mark Theoharis

*5 Child Access Prevention Laws hold gun owners accountable for the safe storage of firearms, imposing liability for failing to take simple yet important measures to prevent guns from falling into young hands. Gifford Law Center http://lawcenter.giffords.org/gun-laws/policy-areas/child-consumer-safety/child-access-prevention/

*6 Blood Loss is what kills most people in this instance. Try to control [bleeding] by applying manual pressure on the wound, or by fastening a

tourniquet high and tight on the limb where the wound is located. What Happens When You Get Shot and How to Survive It

Patrick Allan https://lifehacker.com/what-happens-when-you-get-shot-and-how-to-survive-it-

*7 same source as # 1

*8 Same source as # 2

*9 A seventeen-year-old brought a loaded gun and ammo to school. He will be charged as an adult. May 2018 Rockridge, Florida https://cbs12.com/news/local/teen-found-with-gun-at-school-to-face-charges-as-adult

*10 Crimes committed by children younger than seventeen are called "delinquent acts." If detained in custody, Juvenile court must have a detention hearing within 48 hours of child's arrest. AVVO Attorney Muneer Othman Awad—Legal Guide 10 Things Every Teen Should Know About Juvenile Court

*11 Juvenile Court has the discretion to transfer your case to adult court if they determine you cannot be rehabilitated by the Department of Juvenile Justice.

Muneer Othman Awad—Criminal Defense Attorney—Legal Guide 10 Things Every Teen Should Know About Juvenile Court

*12 Negligent Discharge of a Firearm

Willful discharge of a firearm, in a grossly negligent manner, which could result in someone's injury or death. Examples: After his favorite team won the World Series, a man fired his gun into the air in a park. A 12-year-old boy found a loaded gun which belonged to his father and decided to have target practice by shooting at toys in a room where his younger sister was playing. —Shouse California Law Group

*13 Detention. A juvenile convicted of a weapons possession offense can also be ordered into a group home, juvenile detention center, weekend detention program, a summer "boot camp" program, or other form of detention. Juvenile Weapons Possession By Mark Theoharis

*14. Same source as # 4

*15 Crimes committed by children younger than 17 are called "delinquent acts" and if you are found delinquent, a Juvenile Court judge has the authority to sentence you to confinement and/or supervision until you are 21 years old. Muneer Othman Awad—Criminal Defense Attorney

*16 Reckless endangerment occurs when an individual commits an act recklessly that creates a significant risk of harm, either death or serious bodily injury, to a specific person or persons.

An individual acts recklessly when he does not exercise caution. The individual does not need to intend to harm anyone. legalmatch.com/law-library/article/reckless-endangerment-of-a-child.html

*17 Parents are often accountable for their child's actions. They may be responsible for a child's damages resulting from criminal actions such as vandalism. Parents can also be criminally liable if they "contributed to the delinquency of a minor." An example of this occurs when a child brings a parent's firearm to school, particularly when the parent failed to store the firearm in accordance with state laws. Findlaw.com https://education.findlaw.com/school-safety/weapons-at-school.html

*18 Detention—Same source as #13

*19 Same source as # 12 plus Civil actions could be taken for the injury or death of a pet– Individuals may sue for medical expenses and pain and suffering. The court may award a pet owner punitive damages in cases where the defendant's behavior was excessively negligent. The Law Firm of Aaron A. Herbert, P.C.

*20 Same source as #1

*21 same source as #17

*22 A gunshot that went off in a Los Angeles middle school classroom on Thursday, hitting two students, was accidentally discharged from inside a girl's backpack, Los Angeles police said Friday. A 12-year-old girl was booked on a charge of negligent discharge of a firearm after the shooting, police said. By Andrew Blankstein, Elizabeth Chuck and associated press. discharged in

*23 Possession means both physically carrying a weapon on you and having a weapon in an area that is under your control. This could mean that the weapon was stored in a locker and the student is away from the locker at the time.   Juvenile Weapons Possession By Mark Theoharis

*24 Under the Gun Free School Zones Act of 1995, a firearm could not be brought within 1,000 feet of a school. But the unfortunate reality is that weapons have shown up in our nation's school campuses far too often. https://education.findlaw.com/school-safety/weapons-at-school.html. Forty-seven states and the District of Columbia prohibit carrying or possessing a firearm on K–12 school property, within the safe school or gun-free school zones, on school-provided transportation, or at school-sponsored events. Forty states also ban conceal and carry in their K-12 schools. There are other common exceptions for carrying a gun on school property. Consistent with the federal Gun-Free Schools Act, almost all states expel students for no less than one year for gun possession. To find out the laws in your state or to read common exceptions, go to https://lawcenter.giffords.org/gun-laws/policy-areas/guns-in-public/guns-in-schools/.

*25 A former high school student was sentenced to prison Monday for bringing a loaded firearm to school. Mar'yo Lindsey Jr. was sentenced to five years in prison for carrying weapons, five years for being in possession of a firearm as a felon and two years in prison being in possession of a firearm on school grounds. The sentences are to be served concurrently. Teen gets prison for bringing gun to school JOHN MOLSEED john.molseed@wcfcourier.com Apr 28, 2014

* 26 Students at Oakdale alerted school officials after seeing videos of Robert Antoine Shirley Jr., 18, posing with the weapon on Snapchat.

Shirley was handcuffed, and his jacket and backpack were seized by deputies. The gun was found in his jacket, according to previous reports.

Shirley was charged as an adult because he faced felony charges and had several prior contacts with the juvenile justice system. The legal age to possess a handgun in Maryland is 21.

Student gets 5-year sentence after bringing loaded gun to Oakdale High School By Jeremy Arias jarias@newspost.com

*27 Same source as #1

*28 Same source as #15 and #4

*29 Police can question anyone briefly, including a minor without a Miranda warning. This is known as "Terry Stop." This is legal if an officer has a reasonable suspicion of criminal activity. This is while a kid isn't under arrest and is still free to go. As soon as an arrest is made, the officer must read the Miranda Rights. Shouse Law, Juvenile Interrogation

* 30 Once a police officer arrests a juvenile, he must read them their Miranda Rights, even if he never asks them another question. You have the right to remain silent. Anything you say can and will be used against you in a court of law. You have the right to an attorney. If you cannot afford an attorney, one will be provided for you.

Police Interrogation and Constitutional Miranda Rights in California-- Shouse Law

*31 Same source as number 30

*32 Same source as number 6

* 33 Same source as number 30

* 34 Same source as # 6

* 35 Same as source #3

*36 Same source as # 12

* 37 Same source as # 2

* 38 Same source as # 2

*39 Same source as #1

*40 Same source as #16

*41 Same source as #30

About the Author

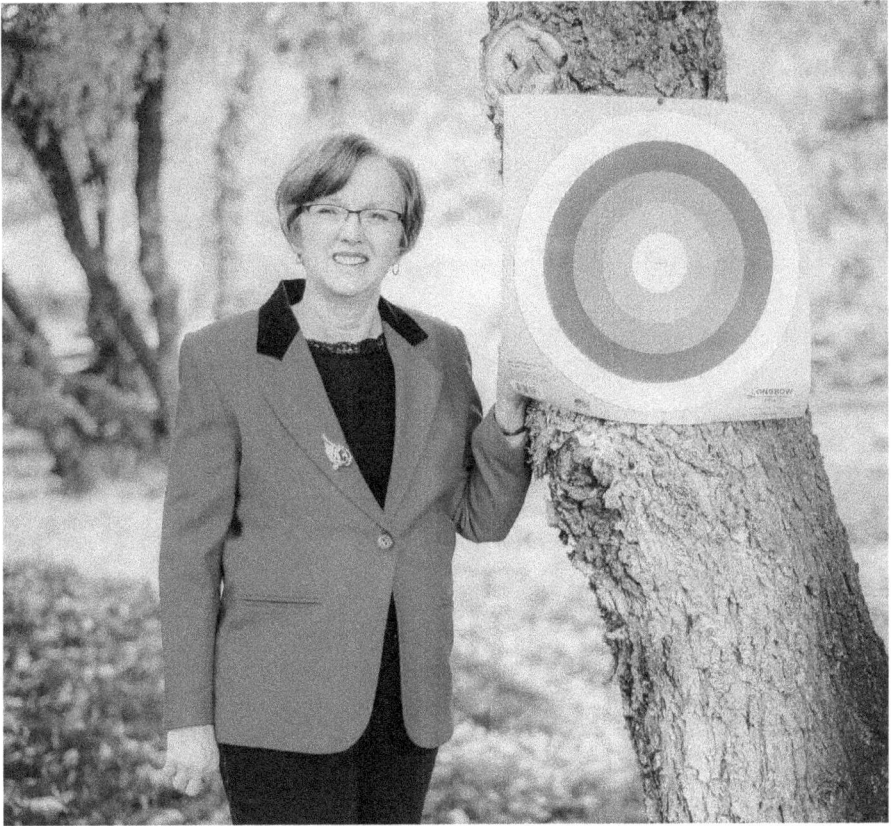

Jill Ammon Vanderwood is the author of ten books for children and young adults. She is the 2008 Writer of the Year from the League of Utah Writers and the winner of numerous book awards, including the National Mom's Choice Award. Jill is making a difference for the next generation by tackling the hard topics affecting kids and their families around our nation, such as drugs, bullying and now gun safety.

In her latest book, Off Target: The Path You Choose # 1, Jill deals in a no-nonsense way with the need for guns to be stored safely away from minors.

About the Illustrators

Kerah Diez is a Utah based artist, working with illustrations and graphics since 2006. She is of Peruvian decent and grew up with an appreciation for traditional and modern art of different countries and cultures. Her appreciation for culture and art led her to study abroad in Japan. This experience has had a great influence on her art pieces today.

Kerah has created illustrations for the Ogden Standard Examiner, newspaper, sticker graphics for the LINE app, children's book illustrations, animations and many other creative projects. She is the illustrator for the Jill Ammon Vanderwood's Christmas books: Santa's Mysterious Boot and The Year Santa Lost His List.

Kerah Diez is well versed in a variety of traditional media, including oil, acrylic and watercolor paints, although most of her work is now digital paintings and graphic design. Kerah can be found on Instagram@kyu10art or at http://kyu10official.wixsite.com/website

Trevor Brown first discovered his talent as an artist while in the first grade, when he drew a boa constrictor with intricate patterns. Throughout his school years, Trevor studied art on his own and took after school art programs. In high school he won Best of Show and Viewer's Choice award in art competitions at local and state fairs.

Trevor served two tours of duty in the U.S. Army, serving in South Korea and Afghanistan. With an honorable discharge from the Army, he began working toward his bachelor's degree in Media Arts and Animation at the Art Institute of Salt Lake City and recently transferred to the Art Institute of Seattle.

Trevor is the illustrator for the covers of Jill Ammon Vanderwood's Through the Rug series and the inside illustrations for Through the Rug 3: Charm Forrest.